Eleanor Greene

The Complete Guide to DIY Natural Skincare

From Beginner to Expert

www.craftyourbetterself.com

To all the women, young and mature, who seek to connect with themselves and the earth through the simple act of caring for their skin—this book is for you. May it guide you on your journey to radiant, healthy skin and a deeper connection with the natural world.

"Let the beauty of what you love be what you do"

— **Rumi,** Persian poet and mystic

TABLE OF CONTENTS

<u>Chapter 10</u>

Sharing Your Passion for Natural Skincare   218

Introduction

Your Journey to Healthy, Radiant Skin

We invite you to embark on a transformative exploration of your skin and the world of natural skincare. Whether you're a skincare novice seeking to revitalize your beauty routine or a seasoned enthusiast eager to deepen your knowledge, this book is your ultimate companion to crafting personalized skincare solutions that nourish, rejuvenate, and empower.

In today's bustling beauty industry, the allure of radiant, healthy skin is undeniable. Yet, amidst the myriad of commercial products promising miraculous results, it's easy to feel overwhelmed and disconnected from the ingredients we're applying to our skin daily. That's where DIY natural skincare steps in—a holistic approach that empowers you to take control of your skincare journey, from formulation to application.

At the heart of DIY natural skincare lies a profound understanding of ingredients—a journey of discovery that goes beyond skincare labels to unveil the true essence of what we're putting on our skin. By delving into the properties, benefits, and origins of natural botanicals, essential oils, and nourishing extracts, we not only gain insight into their transformative powers but also cultivate a deeper connection to nature and our own well-being.

The benefits of embracing DIY natural skincare are manifold. Beyond the allure of crafting luxurious potions and lotions in the comfort of your own home, DIY skincare offers a pathway to empowerment, personalization, and sustainability. By understanding the ingredients that comprise our skincare products, we reclaim the power to tailor formulations to our unique skin types, concerns, and preferences. We liberate ourselves from the constraints of mass-produced beauty standards and embark on a journey of self-discovery and self-care.

Moreover, DIY natural skincare is a testament to environmental stewardship—a conscious choice to embrace eco-friendly practices and reduce our carbon footprint. By opting for sustainably sourced ingredients, minimal packaging, and reusable containers, we not only nourish our skin but also honor our planet, fostering a harmonious relationship with nature that extends far beyond our skincare routines.

As we delve into the chapters ahead, we invite you to embrace the beauty of simplicity, creativity, and authenticity. Whether you're mixing up a nourishing face mask, crafting a rejuvenating serum, or sharing your skincare journey with others, remember that DIY natural skincare is more than just a beauty regimen—it's a celebration of self-love, empowerment, and the timeless wisdom of nature.

So, let's embark on this journey together—to discover the radiant beauty that lies within, to nurture our skin and soul with the bounty of the earth, and to embrace the transformative power of DIY natural skincare. Your journey to healthy, radiant skin starts now.

Chapter 1

Getting Started
with DIY Natural Skincare

Have you ever dreamt of stepping into a world where beauty isn't dictated by potions promising transformation, but by the wisdom to understand what goes into those potions themselves? Imagine yourself on the cusp of an enchanted forest, not armed with a magic wand, but with the knowledge to decipher the ancient scrolls of skincare ingredients. This, dear reader, is the realm of DIY natural skincare, and the key that unlocks its gate is empowerment through knowledge.

Within the labyrinthine world of beauty products, shrouded in promises and marketing sorcery, unraveling the mysteries hidden on product labels becomes an act of liberation. No longer are you at the mercy of misleading claims and empty bottles. With each ingredient you decipher, you reclaim a piece of your skincare routine, shaping it to reflect your desires and understanding your skin's unique language.

This journey of self-discovery extends beyond simply swapping store-bought products for DIY concoctions. It's about personalization – the art of crafting skincare solutions that sing to the symphony of your individual needs. Gone are the days of one-size-fits-all solutions. Here, you become a skilled alchemist, wielding natural ingredients to create personalized elixirs, each one a reflection of your deepest beauty aspirations. With every drop you apply, you weave a tapestry of self-care that speaks to your soul and nourishes your spirit.

But the transformative power of DIY natural skincare extends beyond the confines of your vanity. As you navigate this enchanted forest, you become acutely aware of the impact your choices have on the world around you. Eco-friendly packaging and sustainable ingredient sourcing become a testament to your commitment to the greater good. You realize that true empowerment stems not from selfish indulgence, but from the conscious awareness of your place within the web of life.

Armed with this newfound knowledge and the power of personalization, you venture forth into the unknown, a beacon of light in a world shrouded in commercial gimmicks. With every step you take, you leave behind a legacy of empowerment, self-discovery, and a redefined understanding of beauty. And as you reach the end of this enchanted forest, you realize that the greatest magic lies not in the potions you concoct, but in the transformation that occurs within your heart and soul.

1.1

Benefits of Making
Your Own Skincare Products

Empowerment through Knowledge
Taking Control of Your Beauty Routine

In the ethereal realm of beauty, where potions and elixirs whisper promises of transformation, lies a path to empowerment unlike any other: knowledge. Picture yourself standing at the threshold of this enchanted forest, armed not with a magic wand, but with the wisdom to understand exactly what goes into your skincare products. As you step forward, you embark on a journey of self-discovery and empowerment, where the secrets of skincare ingredients unveil themselves like ancient scrolls, waiting to be deciphered.

Knowledge is the key that unlocks the gates to empowerment. By unraveling the mysteries hidden within skincare labels, you gain a newfound understanding of the potions that grace your vanity. No longer are you at the mercy of marketing sorcery or bewitched by false promises—instead, you hold the reins of control firmly in your hands. With each ingredient you decipher, you take a step closer to reclaiming your beauty routine and shaping it according to your desires.

As you delve deeper into this mystical realm, you discover the power of personalization. Like a skilled alchemist, you learn to tailor your skincare formulations to suit your unique skin type, concerns, and preferences. Gone are the days of one-size-fits-all solutions—

now, you craft potions infused with intention, each one a reflection of your innermost desires and aspirations. With every drop of serum or dollop of cream, you weave a tapestry of self-care that speaks to your soul and nourishes your spirit.

But empowerment through knowledge extends beyond the confines of your skincare routine—it seeps into every aspect of your being, enriching your life in ways you never imagined. As you gaze into the mirror, you see not just a reflection, but a canvas waiting to be adorned with the colors of your choosing. With the wisdom you have gained, you embrace the beauty of imperfection and celebrate the uniqueness of your skin, flaws and all.

Moreover, as you navigate this enchanted forest of beauty, you become acutely aware of the impact your choices have on the world around you. With each eco-friendly packaging choice and sustainable ingredient selection, you leave behind a trail of stardust, a testament to your commitment to the greater good. You realize that true empowerment comes not from selfish indulgence, but from the conscious awareness of your place within the web of life.

And so, armed with the knowledge of skincare ingredients and the power of personalization, you journey forth into the unknown, a beacon of light in a world shrouded in darkness. With each step you take, you leave behind a legacy—a legacy of empowerment, of self-discovery, and of beauty redefined. And as you reach the end of this enchanted forest, you realize that the greatest magic of all lies not in the potions you concoct, but in the transformation that occurs within your heart and soul.

The Art of Personalization
Crafting Solutions for Your Unique Needs

Personalization in skincare refers to the practice of tailoring skincare formulations to suit the specific needs, concerns, and preferences of individuals. It encompasses a holistic approach to skincare that recognizes the diversity of skin types and conditions, as well as the unique preferences and lifestyle choices of each individual. By customizing skincare formulations, individuals can optimize the efficacy and enjoyment of their skincare routines, ultimately achieving healthier, more radiant skin.

At the core of personalization in skincare is the understanding that no two individuals have the same skin. Factors such as genetics, environment, lifestyle, and age all influence the condition and needs of the skin. Personalization acknowledges these differences and seeks to address them through tailored skincare solutions that are specifically formulated to target individual concerns and goals.

One key aspect of personalization is identifying and understanding one's unique skin type. Skin types can vary widely, ranging from dry and sensitive to oily and acne-prone, as well as combination skin types that exhibit characteristics of multiple types. By accurately determining one's skin type, individuals can select skincare products and ingredients that are best suited to their skin's specific needs and requirements.

In addition to skin type, personalization in skincare also involves addressing specific skin concerns. Whether it's acne, aging, hyperpigmentation, or sensitivity, individuals may have specific skincare goals they wish to address. Personalization allows for the selection of ingredients and formulations that target these concerns effectively, helping to improve the overall health and appearance of the skin.

Furthermore, personalization extends beyond addressing skin concerns to encompass individual preferences and lifestyle choices. Some individuals may prefer natural or organic skincare products, while others may prioritize products that are fragrance-free or vegan-friendly. Personalization allows individuals to choose skincare formulations that align with their values and preferences, enhancing their overall skincare experience.

The process of personalization in skincare often involves experimentation and customization. Individuals may need to try out different products and ingredients to find what works best for their skin. DIY skincare recipes and formulations can be particularly useful in this regard, as they allow individuals to control the ingredients used and tailor formulations to their specific needs and preferences.

Personalization in skincare is a fundamental aspect of achieving healthy, radiant skin. By tailoring skincare formulations to suit individual skin types, concerns, and preferences, individuals can optimize the efficacy and enjoyment of their skincare routines. Whether through selecting products off the shelf or experimenting with DIY formulations, personalization empowers individuals to take control of their skincare and achieve their desired results.

Unlocking Beauty on a Budget
The Cost-Effectiveness of DIY Skincare

Achieving radiant, glowing skin doesn't have to come with a hefty price tag. With the rise of DIY skincare, savvy beauty enthusiasts are discovering the art of crafting high-quality products at home using affordable, natural ingredients. In this article, we explore the cost-effectiveness of DIY skincare and how it's revolutionizing the beauty industry.

Gone are the days of splurging on expensive serums and creams—DIY skincare offers a budget-friendly alternative that doesn't compromise on quality. By harnessing the power of nature's bounty, individuals can create customized skincare formulations tailored to their unique needs and preferences, all while saving a pretty penny in the process.

Crafting skincare products at home allows for full control over the ingredients used, ensuring that only the safest and most effective components make their way into your beauty routine. From nourishing oils and butters to soothing botanical extracts and essential oils, the possibilities are endless. Best of all, these natural ingredients can often be sourced affordably from local markets or bulk suppliers, making DIY skincare accessible to all.

But the benefits of DIY skincare go beyond just saving money—it's also a more sustainable choice for both your wallet and the planet. By reducing reliance on commercially packaged products and single-use plastics, individuals can minimize their environmental footprint and contribute to a greener beauty routine. Choosing natural ingredients further supports sustainable farming practices and reduces the environmental impact associated with synthetic chemicals.

Moreover, DIY skincare allows for customization to suit individual skin types and concerns. Whether you're dealing with dryness, acne, or sensitivity, there's a DIY solution for you. From hydrating masks to clarifying toners, the power to tailor your skincare routine lies in your hands, giving you the freedom to address your specific needs effectively.

Crafting skincare products at home can also be a fun and educational experience. Experimenting with different ingredients and formulations allows individuals to gain valuable insight into skincare science and develop a deeper understanding of their skin's needs. Plus, there's something deeply satisfying about creating your own beauty essentials—it's a form of self-expression and empowerment that goes beyond just skincare.

DIY skincare is a game-changer for beauty enthusiasts looking to achieve glowing skin on a budget. By embracing the cost-effectiveness of DIY formulations, individuals can unlock the secrets to radiant skin without breaking the bank. So why not roll up your sleeves, get creative in the kitchen, and embark on a journey to skincare bliss? Your wallet—and your skin—will thank you for it.

Green Beauty
Making a Difference with Eco-Friendly Skincare

As sustainability is becoming increasingly important, eco-conscious beauty enthusiasts are finding new ways to reduce their environmental footprint while still indulging in luxurious skincare routines. Enter the realm of green beauty, where individuals can make a positive impact on the planet by opting for eco-friendly packaging and sustainable ingredient choices.

Environmental impact is a critical consideration in the world of skincare, as traditional beauty products often come with a hefty environmental cost. From single-use plastic packaging to ingredients sourced through unsustainable practices, the beauty industry has historically been a contributor to environmental degradation. However, green beauty offers a solution—a way to enjoy skincare rituals guilt-free while minimizing harm to the planet.

One of the key pillars of green beauty is eco-friendly packaging. By choosing products packaged in recyclable, biodegradable, or reusable materials, individuals can significantly reduce their carbon footprint. From glass bottles and jars to paper or bamboo packaging, there are plenty of sustainable options available that help minimize waste and pollution.

But it's not just about the packaging—sustainable ingredient choices also play a crucial role in reducing environmental impact. Green beauty brands prioritize ingredients that are ethically sourced, sustainably harvested, and environmentally friendly. This means opting for natural, plant-based ingredients that are grown and harvested using eco-friendly practices, such as organic farming or wildcrafting.

Moreover, sustainable ingredient choices extend beyond just the environmental impact—they also offer benefits for both skin health and overall well-being. Natural ingredients are often rich in vitamins, minerals, and antioxidants that nourish and protect the skin, promoting a healthy, radiant complexion without the need for harsh chemicals or synthetic additives.

By embracing green beauty practices, individuals can make a meaningful contribution to environmental conservation while still enjoying the benefits of a luxurious skincare routine. Whether it's choosing products with eco-friendly packaging or selecting formulations made with sustainable ingredients, every small decision adds up to make a positive impact on the planet.

Green beauty is more than just a trend—it's a movement towards a more sustainable and ethical approach to skincare. By reducing our reliance on single-use plastics, opting for recyclable packaging, and choosing products made with sustainably sourced ingredients, we can all do our part to protect the planet and preserve its beauty for future generations.

The Joy of DIY Skincare
Unleashing Creativity and Fun

Within the realm of skincare, DIY formulations serve as a gateway to both creativity and enjoyment, transforming the mundane task of skincare into a fulfilling and engaging hobby. This facet of skincare embraces the spirit of experimentation and exploration, allowing individuals to delve into the world of natural ingredients and formulations with zeal and excitement.

At the core of DIY skincare lies the opportunity for individuals to revel in the creative process, as they blend together a plethora of natural elements to concoct their personalized skincare solutions. From botanical extracts and essential oils to nourishing butters and exfoliating grains, the possibilities for formulation are vast and varied, inviting individuals to exercise their imagination and ingenuity.

The allure of DIY skincare extends beyond mere utility—it offers a source of joy and satisfaction as individuals engage in the hands-on process of crafting their own skincare products. The act of mixing and blending ingredients becomes an artistic endeavor, providing a sense of fulfillment and accomplishment as individuals witness their creations come to life before their eyes.

Moreover, DIY skincare serves as a platform for exploration and discovery, allowing individuals to delve into the intricate world of skincare science and ingredient functionality. Through experimentation with different formulations and techniques, individuals gain valuable insight into the properties of natural ingredients and their effects on the skin, fostering a deeper understanding and appreciation for the art of skincare.

In essence, creativity and fun are at the heart of DIY skincare, offering individuals a means of personal expression and self-discovery within the realm of beauty. By embracing the joy of experimentation and the satisfaction of crafting their own skincare formulations, individuals embark on a journey of empowerment and enrichment, where the pursuit of personalized beauty becomes an enriching and fulfilling endeavor.

1.2

Understanding Labels: Navigating the World of Ingredients

Decoding Skincare Labels
Know Ingredients, Choose With Power

Navigating the vast array of skincare products can often feel like deciphering a complex code, with ingredient lists serving as the key to understanding what goes into each bottle or jar. In this guide, we'll delve into the world of skincare labels, providing practical examples to help you decode ingredient lists and make informed purchasing decisions.

Let's start with a common skincare product: a moisturizing cream. Upon glancing at the ingredient list, you may notice that water (aqua) is listed as the first ingredient. This indicates that water makes up the largest portion of the product, serving as the primary solvent and base. Following water, you might find ingredients like glycerin, a humectant that attracts moisture to the skin, and shea butter, an emollient that helps to soften and smooth the skin's surface.

Now, let's consider a facial cleanser. As you scan the ingredient list, you may come across surfactants such as sodium lauryl sulfate or sodium cocoyl isethionate. These ingredients help to remove dirt, oil, and impurities from the skin by creating a lather. However, some individuals may find these surfactants too harsh or drying, especially if they have sensitive skin. In this case, you might opt for a cleanser formulated with gentler surfactants or natural alternatives like coconut-derived cleansers.

Moving on to a serum targeted at brightening dark spots and hyperpigmentation, you might encounter ingredients like vitamin C (ascorbic acid) and niacinamide (vitamin B3). Both of these ingredients are known for their brightening and skin-evening properties, making them effective choices for addressing hyperpigmentation. Additionally, you may find botanical extracts such as licorice root or mulberry extract, which also have skin-brightening benefits.

Finally, let's explore a sunscreen product. When examining the ingredient list, you'll want to look for broad-spectrum UV filters like zinc oxide or titanium dioxide, which provide protection against both UVA and UVB rays. Additionally, you may find antioxidants such as vitamin E or green tea extract, which help to neutralize free radicals generated by UV exposure and minimize oxidative damage to the skin.

Decoding skincare labels is a valuable skill that empowers consumers to make informed choices about the products they use on their skin. By understanding the function and purpose of common skincare ingredients and paying attention to potential allergens or irritants, individuals can navigate the world of skincare with confidence, ensuring they select products that align with their unique needs and preferences.

Steering Clear of Harmful Ingredients
A Guide to Identifying Common Skincare Culprits

In the pursuit of healthy, radiant skin, it's essential to be mindful of the ingredients lurking in the products we use daily. While many skincare products promise transformative results, some may contain harmful ingredients that can irritate the skin, trigger allergies, or even pose long-term health risks. In this guide, we'll shine a light on some common culprits to watch out for in commercial skincare products, empowering you to make informed choices for your skin's well-being.

Parabens: Widely used as preservatives to extend the shelf life of skincare products, parabens have come under scrutiny due to their potential hormone-disrupting properties. Commonly listed as methylparaben, ethylparaben, propylparaben, and butylparaben, these ingredients may mimic estrogen in the body and have been linked to hormonal imbalances and reproductive issues.

Sulfates: Surfactants like sodium lauryl sulfate (SLS) and sodium laureth sulfate (SLES) are frequently used in cleansers and shampoos for their foaming properties. However, these harsh detergents can strip the skin of its natural oils, leading to dryness, irritation, and disruption of the skin barrier. Individuals with sensitive or dry skin may be particularly prone to adverse reactions from sulfates.

Fragrance: While a pleasant scent may enhance the sensory experience of skincare products, synthetic fragrances can be a hidden source of irritation and allergens. Fragrance blends often contain a cocktail of potentially harmful chemicals, including phthalates, which have been linked to hormone disruption and allergic reactions. Opting for fragrance-free or products scented with natural essential oils can help minimize the risk of irritation.

Mineral Oil: Derived from petroleum, mineral oil is a common ingredient in moisturizers and ointments due to its occlusive properties, which help to lock in moisture. However, mineral oil forms a barrier on the skin's surface that can clog pores and prevent the skin from breathing, potentially leading to breakouts and exacerbating acne-prone skin.

Formaldehyde-Releasing Preservatives: Certain preservatives, such as diazolidinyl urea, imidazolidinyl urea, and DMDM hydantoin, release formaldehyde over time to prevent microbial growth in skincare products. Formaldehyde is a known carcinogen and skin irritant, posing health risks with prolonged exposure. Choosing products formulated with alternative preservatives or opting for preservative-free formulations can help minimize exposure to formaldehyde.

By familiarizing yourself with these common harmful ingredients and reading skincare labels with a discerning eye, you can take proactive steps to avoid potential irritants, allergens, and toxins in your skincare products. Prioritizing products formulated with safe and gentle ingredients can help maintain the health and vitality of your skin, allowing you to achieve your skincare goals while minimizing the risk of adverse reactions.

Spotlight on Natural Ingredients
Harnessing the Power of Botanicals

Nature has long been revered for its ability to nourish, heal, and rejuvenate the skin. From time-honored botanicals to aromatic essential oils, natural ingredients offer a wealth of benefits for skin health and beauty. In this spotlight, we'll explore the wonders of natural botanicals, essential oils, and plant-based extracts, uncovering their transformative potential for achieving radiant, youthful-looking skin.

Botanicals: Derived from plants, botanical ingredients are packed with vitamins, antioxidants, and nutrients that can help promote skin health and vitality. Common botanicals like aloe vera, chamomile, and calendula are prized for their soothing and anti-inflammatory properties, making them ideal for calming sensitive or irritated skin. Additionally, botanical extracts such as green tea, licorice root, and rosehip oil boast potent antioxidant benefits, helping to protect the skin from environmental damage and premature aging.

Essential Oils: Aromatic and potent, essential oils are prized for their therapeutic properties and aromatic benefits. These concentrated plant extracts are rich in bioactive compounds that can address a wide range of skin concerns, from acne and blemishes to dryness and aging. Lavender essential oil, for example, is renowned for its calming and balancing properties, making it a popular choice for promoting relaxation and soothing irritated skin. Meanwhile, tea tree oil is prized for its antibacterial and anti-inflammatory properties, making it an effective treatment for acne-prone skin.

Plant-Based Extracts: Extracts derived from fruits, flowers, and herbs offer a concentrated dose of botanical goodness, delivering targeted benefits for specific skin concerns. For example, grape seed extract is rich in antioxidants like proanthocyanidins, which help protect the skin from free radical damage and support collagen production, leading to firmer, more youthful-looking skin. Similarly, cucumber extract is known for its hydrating and cooling properties, making it a refreshing addition to skincare products designed to soothe and hydrate the skin.

Natural ingredients offer a treasure trove of benefits for skin health and beauty, harnessing the power of botanicals, essential oils, and plant-based extracts to nourish, protect, and rejuvenate the skin. Whether you're looking to soothe sensitive skin, combat signs of aging, or simply pamper yourself with the goodness of nature, incorporating natural ingredients into your skincare routine can help you achieve the radiant, glowing complexion you've always desired.

Allergen Awareness
Protecting Sensitive Skin from Potential Irritants

Achieving healthy and radiant skin often involves navigating through a maze of products, each promising transformative results. However, for individuals with sensitive skin, this journey can be fraught with challenges, as certain ingredients have the potential to trigger adverse reactions and exacerbate existing skin concerns. In this guide, we'll shed light on the importance of allergen awareness and highlight common allergens and sensitizing ingredients to watch out for in skincare products.

Fragrances: While the scent of a skincare product can be enticing, fragrances are among the most common culprits for skin irritation and allergic reactions. Synthetic fragrances, in particular, often contain a cocktail of potentially irritating chemicals, such as phthalates and synthetic musks, which can wreak havoc on sensitive skin. Opting for fragrance-free or products scented with natural essential oils can help minimize the risk of irritation and allergic reactions.

Preservatives: Preservatives play a crucial role in preventing microbial growth and extending the shelf life of skincare products. However, certain preservatives, such as parabens and formaldehyde-releasing agents, have been associated with allergic reactions and skin sensitization. Individuals with sensitive skin may be particularly susceptible to these preservatives, leading to redness, itching, and inflammation. Choosing products formulated with alternative preservatives or opting for preservative-free formulations can help reduce the risk of adverse reactions.

Common Allergens: Certain ingredients commonly found in skincare products have the potential to trigger allergic reactions in sensitive individuals. These include but are not limited to, lanolin, a wool-derived ingredient often found in moisturizers and lip balms, and certain botanical extracts such as chamomile and lavender, which can cause contact dermatitis in some individuals. Patch testing new products before full application can help identify potential allergens and prevent adverse reactions.

Harsh Surfactants: Surfactants like sodium lauryl sulfate (SLS) and sodium laureth sulfate (SLES) are commonly used in cleansers and body washes for their foaming properties. However, these harsh detergents can strip the skin of its natural oils and disrupt the skin barrier, leading to dryness, irritation, and inflammation, particularly in individuals with sensitive skin. Opting for gentle cleansers formulated with mild surfactants or natural alternatives can help minimize the risk of irritation.

Allergen awareness is essential for individuals with sensitive skin to protect against potential irritants and allergens in skincare products. By avoiding common allergens and sensitizing ingredients, patch testing new products, and opting for gentle formulations designed for sensitive skin, individuals can reduce the risk of adverse reactions and maintain a healthy and comfortable complexion.

1.3

Setting Up
Your Skincare Workspace

A Clean and Organized Environment
Elevating Your Skincare Ritual

Carving out moments of tranquility and self-care is essential for maintaining balance and well-being. Amidst the chaos of daily life, our skincare routine offers a sanctuary—a moment of solace and rejuvenation. Designating a dedicated area in your home for skincare formulation is more than just a practical measure; it's a transformative step towards enhancing your beauty ritual and reclaiming a sense of calm amidst the chaos.

First and foremost, creating a clean and organized environment for skincare formulation sets the stage for a seamless and enjoyable experience. By designating a specific area in your home, whether it's a corner of your bedroom, a cozy nook in the living room, or a dedicated vanity space, you establish a dedicated sanctuary where you can focus solely on your skincare routine without distractions.

A clutter-free environment is not just visually pleasing—it's conducive to creativity and clarity of mind. Decluttering your skincare space and organizing your tools and products in an orderly fashion not only streamlines your routine but also enhances efficiency and reduces stress. With everything in its rightful place, you can navigate your skincare ritual with ease, free from the frustration of searching for misplaced items or dealing with cluttered countertops.

Investing in proper storage solutions is essential for maintaining the integrity and efficacy of your skincare products. Glass jars, airtight containers, and labeled organizers not only add a touch of sophistication to your space but also ensure that your products remain fresh and protected from light, heat, and moisture. By treating your skincare ingredients with care and respect, you elevate your beauty ritual to a luxurious and indulgent experience.

Optimizing your skincare environment goes beyond aesthetics—it's about creating a sensory oasis that engages all the senses. Soft lighting, soothing music, and aromatic candles infuse your space with a sense of tranquility and relaxation, transforming your skincare routine into a luxurious self-care ritual. By engaging the senses, you deepen your connection to the present moment and cultivate a sense of mindfulness and well-being.

Creating a clean and organized environment for skincare formulation is a transformative step towards enhancing your beauty ritual and reclaiming a sense of calm amidst the chaos of daily life. By designating a dedicated space, decluttering and organizing your tools and products, investing in proper storage solutions, and infusing your space with sensory delights, you elevate your skincare routine to a luxurious and indulgent experience worthy of the time and attention it deserves.

Equipping Your Skincare Sanctuary
Tools and Ingredients for Crafting Beauty

In the realm of skincare formulation, having the right tools and ingredients at your disposal is essential for creating effective and luxurious formulations. From mixing bowls to high-quality ingredients, each element plays a crucial role in elevating your skincare ritual to new heights. In this guide, we'll explore the essential equipment and supplies you need to stock up on to transform your home into a skincare sanctuary.

Mixing Bowls: A set of mixing bowls is the cornerstone of any skincare formulation workspace. Opt for durable, non-reactive materials like glass or stainless steel, which won't absorb odors or leach chemicals into your formulations. Having multiple sizes on hand allows you to accommodate various batch sizes and ensures you have the flexibility to experiment with different formulations.

Measuring Spoons and Cups: Accurate measurements are key to crafting consistent and effective skincare formulations. Invest in a set of measuring spoons and cups, preferably made from food-grade materials like stainless steel or BPA-free plastic. These tools allow you to precisely measure out ingredients, ensuring that your formulations are balanced and effective.

Storage Containers: Proper storage is essential for preserving the integrity and potency of your skincare ingredients. Stock up on a variety of storage containers, including glass jars, bottles, and tubes, to store your formulations safely and securely. Opt for containers with airtight seals to protect your formulations from light, air, and moisture, prolonging their shelf life and efficacy.

High-Quality Ingredients: The foundation of any skincare formulation is the ingredients you choose to incorporate. Invest in high-quality, ethically sourced ingredients that are suited to your skin type and concerns. Whether you're drawn to botanical extracts, nourishing oils, or potent actives like hyaluronic acid and vitamin C, prioritize ingredients that are backed by scientific research and formulated for maximum efficacy.

Labeling Supplies: Keep your formulations organized and easily identifiable by labeling your containers with the names and dates of your creations. Stock up on waterproof labels and permanent markers to ensure that your labels remain legible and intact, even in humid bathroom environments. Proper labeling not only adds a professional touch to your skincare creations but also helps you track the shelf life of your formulations.

Stocking up on essential equipment and supplies is the first step towards transforming your home into a skincare sanctuary. By investing in quality tools like mixing bowls and measuring spoons, sourcing high-quality ingredients, and ensuring proper storage and labeling of your formulations, you can elevate your skincare ritual to new heights of luxury and efficacy. With the right tools and ingredients at your disposal, you have the power to craft personalized skincare formulations that nourish, rejuvenate, and enhance your natural beauty.

Safety First
Crafting Skincare with Confidence

Ensuring safety is like laying a sturdy foundation before building a beautiful house. It's not just about the end result; it's about the process too. From picking ingredients to handling them, every step matters for your well-being. Let's explore how to navigate this journey safely, without losing any of the fun.

When it comes to handling skincare ingredients, treat them like the precious gems they are. Some ingredients can be potent or irritating if not handled carefully. Always read instructions carefully and wear protective gear like gloves and goggles to shield yourself from any potential hazards.

Equip yourself with the right tools of the trade. Gloves protect your hands from direct contact with ingredients, while goggles shield your eyes from splashes. And hey, why not don a stylish lab coat or apron too? Not only does it keep your clothes clean, but it also adds a touch of professionalism to your setup.

Storing your skincare ingredients properly is key to keeping them fresh and effective. Store them in a cool, dry place away from sunlight and heat. Use airtight containers to prevent air and moisture from sneaking in, and don't forget to label them for easy identification.

If you have little ones or furry friends running around, make sure your ingredients are stored safely out of their reach. Kids and pets are naturally curious, and some ingredients might not be safe for them. So, keep those cabinets locked up tight!

In case of any accidents, having a first aid kit on hand is a life-saver. Stock it with essentials like bandages, antiseptic wipes, and eye wash solution. And make sure you know who to call in an emergency—having poison control's number handy is always a good idea.

In a nutshell, safety is the name of the game in DIY skincare. By taking simple precautions like handling ingredients carefully, using protective gear, storing them properly, and being prepared for emergencies, you can create your skincare creations with confidence. So, roll up your sleeves, put on your gloves, and let's get crafting—safely and stylishly!

Crafting with Care
Practicing Good Manufacturing Practices

Ensuring the safety and efficacy of your creations is paramount. Good Manufacturing Practices (GMP) serve as the guiding principles for maintaining quality, consistency, and safety in skincare formulation. By establishing hygienic practices and adhering to recipe guidelines meticulously, you can create skincare products that are not only effective but also safe for use. Let's delve into the importance of GMP in homemade skincare and how to implement them effectively.

Hygienic Practices: The foundation of GMP lies in maintaining a clean and hygienic environment for skincare formulation. Before diving into the formulation process, ensure that your workspace and equipment are thoroughly sanitized. Wash your hands with soap and water, and disinfect all surfaces and tools to prevent contamination. By prioritizing hygiene, you minimize the risk of introducing harmful bacteria or pathogens into your skincare products.

Sanitizing Equipment: Proper sanitation of equipment is essential for preventing cross-contamination and ensuring product safety. Before each use, sterilize your mixing bowls, utensils, and containers with hot water and soap or a diluted bleach solution. Rinse thoroughly and allow to air dry before proceeding with formulation. Regularly clean and disinfect equipment to maintain a hygienic workspace and prevent the growth of bacteria or mold.

Following Recipe Guidelines: Recipes serve as the blueprint for creating homemade skincare products, providing precise measurements and instructions for each ingredient. When formulating skincare products, it's crucial to follow recipe guidelines meticulously to ensure accurate results and product efficacy. Avoid deviating from the recommended proportions or substituting ingredients unless you have a thorough understanding of their properties and effects on the final product.

Quality Ingredients: In addition to following recipe guidelines, using high-quality ingredients is essential for achieving optimal results in homemade skincare formulations. Choose ingredients that are sourced from reputable suppliers and free from contaminants or adulterants. Prioritize natural, organic ingredients whenever possible, and avoid using expired or compromised ingredients that may compromise the safety and efficacy of your products.

Documentation and Record-Keeping: Keeping thorough documentation of your skincare formulations is essential for maintaining accountability and traceability in the manufacturing process. Record the ingredients used, batch numbers, and dates of formulation for each product to track their shelf life and ensure consistency in quality. By maintaining detailed records, you can identify and address any issues that arise and make informed decisions about product safety and efficacy.

Continuous Improvement: GMP is not a one-time effort but an ongoing commitment to excellence and continuous improvement. Regularly review and evaluate your skincare formulation processes to identify areas for optimization and enhancement. Stay informed about industry best practices and regulatory guidelines to ensure compliance and uphold the highest standards of quality and safety in your homemade skincare products.

Implementing Good Manufacturing Practices is essential for ensuring the safety, efficacy, and quality of homemade skincare products. By establishing hygienic practices, sanitizing equipment, following recipe guidelines meticulously, using quality ingredients, maintaining documentation, and embracing continuous improvement, you can create skincare products that are not only effective but also safe for use. With GMP as your guiding principle, you can craft with care and confidence, knowing that you're prioritizing the well-being of yourself and your customers.

Chapter 2

Know Your Skin: Identifying Your Skin Type and Concerns

The human face is a captivating canvas, and each individual's skin tells a unique story. Unraveling the secrets your skin whispers is the first step towards crafting a personalized DIY skincare routine. This routine becomes your map, guiding you on a journey towards a healthy, radiant complexion that celebrates your skin's specific needs and desires.

Understanding the different landscapes of skin types is paramount. Imagine traversing the balanced plains of normal skin, the delicate valleys of sensitive skin, or the areas prone to dryness or excess oil production - each terrain demands a specific approach. By identifying your skin's unique topography, you unlock a treasure trove of knowledge. You become empowered to select ingredients that speak its specific language, creating a personalized recipe for a healthy and glowing complexion.

Perhaps your skin whispers a tale of dryness, a parched landscape yearning for hydration. Nature's bounty unfolds before you, offering a symphony of nourishing ingredients. Hydrating aloe vera acts like a gentle rain, replenishing moisture. Humectant honey draws in precious water from the air, while emollient shea butter smooths and softens the surface. Each ingredient plays a vital role, composing a personalized blend designed to restore balance and quench your skin's thirst.

On the other hand, your skin might tell a different story, one of excessive oil production. This calls for venturing into the realm of balancing ingredients. Astringent witch hazel acts like a natural stream, gently tightening pores and regulating oil flow. Lightweight grapeseed oil provides essential hydration without tipping the scales towards oiliness. Remember, balance is key, and with each ingredient you choose, you refine your personalized map towards healthy oil control.

But the narrative doesn't end there. Your skin might have additional chapters - chapters that speak of blemishes, hyperpigmentation, or signs of aging. Fear not, for nature's bounty offers solutions for these concerns as well. Anti-inflammatory botanicals can soothe blemishes, calming the landscape. Brightening botanical extracts, like a natural sunrise, can help address hyperpigmentation. And for those seeking to combat the signs of time, antioxidant-rich oils like rosehip seed oil offer a natural defense against free radicals, protecting your skin from the elements.

Unveiling your skin's story is the key to crafting a personalized DIY skincare routine. By deciphering its whispers and understanding its unique needs, you unlock the power to select the perfect ingredients to nurture its health and promote a radiant glow from within. So, embark on this journey of self-discovery, and together, let's create a personalized adventure towards a healthy, radiant complexion that celebrates your skin's unique narrative.

2.1

Skin Types Demystified: Finding Your Skin's Profile

Normal Skin
Embracing the Balance

Normal skin—a coveted state of equilibrium where neither oiliness nor dryness reigns supreme. It's the Goldilocks of skin types, with just the right amount of hydration, minimal sensitivity, and few visible imperfections. In the realm of skincare, understanding the characteristics of normal skin is essential for maintaining its delicate balance and preserving its natural beauty. Let's explore what sets normal skin apart and how to care for it effectively.

Balanced Hydration: Normal skin boasts optimal moisture levels, neither excessively oily nor parched. Its balanced hydration ensures a soft, supple texture and a radiant complexion. Unlike dry skin, which may feel tight and rough, or oily skin, which can appear shiny and prone to breakouts, normal skin strikes the perfect balance, feeling comfortable and hydrated without any greasiness.

Minimal Sensitivity: Normal skin tends to be resilient and tolerant, exhibiting minimal sensitivity to environmental stressors and skincare products. It rarely reacts adversely to new products or ingredients, making it an ideal canvas for experimentation. Unlike sensitive skin, which may experience redness, irritation, or allergic reactions, normal skin maintains its composure, remaining calm and collected even in the face of external aggressors.

Few Visible Imperfections: While no skin type is entirely flawless, normal skin is characterized by its minimal imperfections. It may occasionally experience blemishes or breakouts, but they are typically mild and infrequent. Normal skin has a smooth, even texture with small pores and a healthy complexion. Unlike combination skin, which may exhibit oily and dry areas, normal skin maintains consistency across the entire face.

Caring for Normal Skin: Despite its seemingly effortless beauty, normal skin still requires care and attention to maintain its balance and vitality. A gentle and consistent skincare routine is key to preserving its natural radiance. Cleansing with a mild, pH-balanced cleanser removes impurities without stripping away essential moisture. Follow up with a lightweight moisturizer to hydrate and protect the skin barrier.

Sun Protection: Even normal skin is not immune to the damaging effects of UV radiation. Incorporating a broad-spectrum sunscreen into your daily routine is essential for safeguarding against premature aging, sunburn, and skin cancer. Opt for a lightweight, non-comedogenic formula with an SPF of 30 or higher, and reapply regularly, especially when spending extended periods outdoors.

Regular Exfoliation: While normal skin may not require intensive exfoliation, incorporating gentle exfoliants into your routine can help maintain its smooth texture and clarity. Choose chemical exfoliants like AHAs or BHAs, which gently dissolve dead skin cells and unclog pores without causing irritation. Limit exfoliation to once or twice a week to avoid over-exfoliation and maintain the skin's natural balance.

Balanced Diet and Lifestyle: Lastly, maintaining a balanced diet and lifestyle is crucial for promoting the health and vitality of normal skin. Stay hydrated by drinking plenty of water, eat a nutritious diet rich in fruits, vegetables, and lean proteins, and manage stress levels through relaxation techniques like meditation or yoga. A holistic approach to wellness supports the overall health of normal skin from the inside out.

Normal skin is a testament to balance and harmony—a canvas of beauty that requires care and attention to preserve its natural radiance. By understanding its characteristics and adopting a gentle yet consistent skincare routine, you can embrace the beauty of normal skin and revel in its effortless glow for years to come.

Dry Skin
Nourishing the Thirsty Canvas

Dry skin—the parched desert in the landscape of skin types, often marked by signs of dehydration, flakiness, and tightness. It's a common condition that can be influenced by various factors, including environmental elements and hormonal fluctuations. Understanding the signs of dry skin and its underlying causes is essential for developing an effective skincare regimen to replenish moisture and restore balance. Let's explore the characteristics of dry skin and how to address its needs effectively.

Signs of Dryness: Dry skin is characterized by a lack of moisture, resulting in a dull, rough, and sometimes flaky appearance. It may feel tight or uncomfortable, especially after cleansing or exposure to harsh weather conditions. Unlike normal or oily skin, which maintains a natural balance of oil and moisture, dry skin lacks sufficient hydration, leading to visible signs of dryness and discomfort.

Flakiness and Tightness: One of the telltale signs of dry skin is flakiness, particularly on areas like the cheeks, forehead, and around the nose. The skin may appear dull and lackluster, with visible flakes or patches of dry, rough texture. Additionally, dry skin often feels tight and stretched, especially after washing or prolonged exposure to dry air. This tightness is a result of the skin's inability to retain moisture, leaving it feeling dry and uncomfortable.

Environmental Factors: Environmental factors play a significant role in exacerbating dry skin. Exposure to cold, dry air, harsh winds, and low humidity levels can strip the skin of its natural oils and moisture, leading to increased dryness and sensitivity. Indoor heating during the winter months can further exacerbate the problem, causing moisture loss and dehydration. Additionally, hot showers or baths can strip the skin of its natural oils, exacerbating dryness and exacerbating existing symptoms.

Hormonal Changes: Hormonal fluctuations can also contribute to dry skin, particularly in women. Changes in hormone levels, such as during puberty, pregnancy, or menopause, can affect the skin's ability to retain moisture and regulate oil production. As hormone levels fluctuate, the skin may become drier and more prone to dehydration, leading to increased sensitivity and discomfort.

Addressing Dry Skin: To address dry skin effectively, it's essential to focus on replenishing moisture and restoring the skin's natural barrier function. Incorporating hydrating skincare products rich in emollients, humectants, and occlusives can help lock in moisture and prevent moisture loss. Look for ingredients like hyaluronic acid, glycerin, ceramides, and natural oils, which help nourish and hydrate the skin.

Gentle Cleansing: When cleansing dry skin, opt for gentle, hydrating cleansers that remove impurities without stripping away essential moisture. Avoid harsh soaps or foaming cleansers, which can further deplete the skin's natural oils and exacerbate dryness. Instead, choose creamy or oil-based cleansers that hydrate and nourish the skin while cleansing.

Moisturize Regularly: Moisturizing is a crucial step in any skincare routine, especially for dry skin. Apply a rich, nourishing moisturizer to damp skin immediately after cleansing to lock in moisture and prevent dryness. Look for moisturizers with ingredients like shea butter, jojoba oil, or squalane, which provide intense hydration and improve skin texture and elasticity.

Humidify the Air: To combat the drying effects of indoor heating or dry climates, consider using a humidifier in your home or office. A humidifier adds moisture to the air, helping to maintain optimal humidity levels and prevent excessive moisture loss from the skin. This can help alleviate dryness and discomfort, especially during the winter months.

Protect from Environmental Stressors: Protecting the skin from environmental stressors is essential for preventing further moisture loss and damage. Wear protective clothing, such as scarves or hats, to shield the skin from harsh winds and cold temperatures. Additionally, use a broad-spectrum sunscreen daily to protect against UV radiation, which can further dehydrate and damage dry skin.

Hydrate from Within: In addition to topical skincare products, staying hydrated from within is crucial for maintaining healthy, hydrated skin. Drink plenty of water throughout the day to support skin hydration and overall health. Eating a balanced diet rich in fruits, vegetables, and omega-3 fatty acids can also help nourish the skin from the inside out, promoting hydration and vitality.

Dry skin often shows signs like dehydration, flakiness, and tightness. Knowing its causes and using hydrating skincare can restore moisture and comfort. Hydrating products, gentle cleansing, and protection against environmental stressors nourish dry skin, bringing back its radiance.

Oily Skin
Balancing the Shine

Oily skin—often associated with a persistent shine, enlarged pores, and a predisposition to acne and blackheads. It's a common skin type caused by excess sebum production, which can leave the skin looking greasy and prone to blemishes. Understanding the characteristics of oily skin and how to manage it effectively is essential for achieving a balanced and healthy complexion. Let's delve into the unique features of oily skin and explore strategies for controlling shine and minimizing breakouts.

Excess Sebum Production: Oily skin is characterized by an overproduction of sebum, the skin's natural oil. Sebum plays a crucial role in maintaining skin hydration and protecting against moisture loss. However, when sebum production becomes excessive, it can lead to a shiny, greasy appearance that persists throughout the day. This excess oiliness can contribute to clogged pores, acne, and blackheads, creating an uneven and congested complexion.

Shine and Enlarged Pores: One of the hallmark signs of oily skin is the presence of shine, particularly in the T-zone area (forehead, nose, and chin). This shine is caused by the accumulation of sebum on the skin's surface, giving it a glossy or greasy appearance. Additionally, oily skin often features enlarged pores, which may appear more prominent due to the excess oil production. Enlarged pores are more susceptible to trapping dirt, oil, and impurities, leading to congestion and breakouts.

Propensity for Acne and Blackheads: Oily skin is more prone to acne and blackheads due to the excess sebum production and the buildup of dead skin cells and debris within the pores. The combination of oil, bacteria, and inflammation can lead to the formation of whiteheads, blackheads, pimples, and cysts. Acne breakouts are common on the face, chest, and back—areas where sebaceous glands are most abundant—and can have a significant impact on self-esteem and confidence.

Managing Oily Skin: While oily skin can pose challenges, it is entirely manageable with the right skincare regimen and lifestyle habits. The key is to balance sebum production, control shine, and prevent breakouts without stripping the skin of its natural oils.

Gentle Cleansing: Proper cleansing is essential for removing excess oil, dirt, and impurities from the skin's surface without over-drying or irritating the skin. Opt for gentle, non-comedogenic cleansers that effectively remove oil and debris without stripping the skin's natural moisture barrier. Cleansing twice daily—morning and night—helps keep oil production in check and prevents the buildup of pore-clogging impurities.

Balancing Moisturization: Contrary to popular belief, oily skin still requires hydration to maintain a healthy balance. Choose lightweight, oil-free moisturizers that provide hydration without adding excess oil to the skin. Look for water-based or gel formulations that absorb quickly and leave a matte finish. Moisturizing regularly helps prevent the skin from overcompensating for dryness by producing even more oil.

Exfoliation: Regular exfoliation is essential for removing dead skin cells and unclogging pores, preventing blackheads and acne breakouts. Incorporate exfoliating products containing alpha hydroxy acids (AHAs) or beta hydroxy acids (BHAs) into your skincare routine to promote cell turnover and reveal smoother, clearer skin. However, avoid over-exfoliating, as it can strip the skin's protective barrier and exacerbate oiliness.

Oil-Control Products: Incorporating oil-control products into your skincare routine can help manage shine and reduce excess oil production. Look for products containing ingredients like salicylic acid, niacinamide, or witch hazel, which help regulate sebum production and minimize pore size. Oil-absorbing sheets or blotting papers are also handy for quickly removing excess oil throughout the day without disturbing makeup.

Sun Protection: Don't forget to protect your skin from the sun, even if you have oily skin. Choose lightweight, oil-free sunscreens with a matte finish to prevent sun damage and premature aging. Look for broad-spectrum formulas with an SPF of 30 or higher, and reapply regularly, especially when spending extended periods outdoors.

Healthy Lifestyle Habits: Maintaining a healthy lifestyle can also help manage oily skin. Avoiding excessive sun exposure, minimizing stress, getting enough sleep, and eating a balanced diet rich in fruits, vegetables, and whole grains can all contribute to healthier, more balanced skin.

Oily skin is characterized by excess sebum production, shine, enlarged pores, and a propensity for acne and blackheads. While managing oily skin can be challenging, it is entirely manageable with the right skincare regimen and lifestyle habits. By incorporating gentle cleansing, balancing moisturization, regular exfoliation, oil-control products, sun protection, and healthy lifestyle habits into your routine, you can effectively manage oily skin and achieve a clearer, more balanced complexion.

Combination Skin
Balancing Duality

Combination skin—a blend of contrasts, where oily and dry areas coexist on the same canvas. It's a common skin type characterized by a delicate balance of moisture levels, with oiliness typically concentrated in the T-zone (forehead, nose, and chin) and dryness prevalent in other areas of the face. Understanding the unique characteristics of combination skin and adopting a tailored skincare approach is essential for achieving harmony and maintaining a healthy complexion. Let's delve into the nuances of combination skin and explore strategies for effectively managing its diverse needs.

The Yin and Yang of Combination Skin: Combination skin presents a unique duality, with contrasting characteristics that require specialized care. The T-zone—comprising the forehead, nose, and chin—tends to be oilier due to a higher density of sebaceous glands, while other areas of the face may experience dryness or normal skin conditions. This imbalance in oil production can lead to a variety of skincare concerns, including enlarged pores, shine, dry patches, and occasional breakouts.

Oily T-Zone: The T-zone is the epicenter of oiliness in combination skin, with sebaceous glands in this area producing excess sebum. This can result in a shiny or greasy appearance, enlarged pores, and a predisposition to blackheads and acne. Managing oiliness in the T-zone requires targeted treatments and products designed to regulate sebum production without over-drying the skin or exacerbating dryness in other areas.

Dry or Normal Cheeks: In contrast to the oily T-zone, the cheeks may experience dryness or normal skin conditions in individuals with combination skin. These areas may feel tight, rough, or flaky, especially during colder months or in response to environmental factors like indoor heating or air conditioning. Proper hydration and moisturization are essential for replenishing moisture and restoring balance to dry or normal areas of the face.

Managing Combination Skin: Effectively managing combination skin requires a multifaceted approach that addresses both oily and dry areas without causing further imbalance. Tailoring your skincare routine to target specific concerns in different areas of the face can help achieve a harmonious complexion and minimize the risk of breakouts or irritation.

Gentle Cleansing: Begin your skincare routine with a gentle, non-drying cleanser that effectively removes impurities and excess oil without stripping the skin's natural moisture barrier. Look for pH-balanced formulas that provide a thorough cleanse without causing irritation or dryness. Avoid harsh soaps or foaming cleansers, which can exacerbate dryness in certain areas of the face.

Targeted Treatments: Incorporate targeted treatments into your skincare routine to address the specific needs of different areas of the face. For the oily T-zone, use oil-control products containing ingredients like salicylic acid or niacinamide to regulate sebum production and minimize shine. For dry or normal areas, opt for hydrating serums or moisturizers enriched with nourishing ingredients like hyaluronic acid or ceramides to replenish moisture and restore balance.

Balanced Moisturization: Strike a balance between hydration and oil control by choosing lightweight, oil-free moisturizers that provide hydration without adding excess oil to the skin. Apply moisturizer generously to dry or normal areas of the face, focusing on areas prone to dryness or flakiness, while using a lighter touch in the oily T-zone to prevent shine and congestion.

Sun Protection: Protecting combination skin from the sun is essential for preventing sun damage and premature aging. Choose a broad-spectrum sunscreen with an SPF of 30 or higher that offers protection against UVA and UVB rays. Look for lightweight, non-comedogenic formulas that won't clog pores or exacerbate oiliness in the T-zone.

Balanced Diet and Lifestyle: Maintaining a healthy lifestyle can also contribute to balanced skin. Stay hydrated by drinking plenty of water, eat a balanced diet rich in fruits, vegetables, and omega-3 fatty acids, and manage stress levels through relaxation techniques like meditation or yoga. These lifestyle habits support overall skin health and contribute to a harmonious complexion.

Combination skin presents a unique set of challenges and opportunities, with oily and dry areas coexisting on the same canvas. By understanding the characteristics of combination skin and adopting a tailored skincare approach, you can achieve balance and harmony in your complexion. Incorporate gentle cleansing, targeted treatments, balanced moisturization, sun protection, and healthy lifestyle habits into your routine to effectively manage combination skin and maintain a healthy, radiant complexion.

Sensitive Skin
Navigating Reactivity with Care

Sensitive skin, akin to a finely tuned instrument, reacts swiftly and intensely to external stimuli, displaying telltale signs of redness, itching, and a predisposition to allergic reactions or irritation. Unlike its resilient counterparts, sensitive skin requires a gentle touch and a mindful approach to skincare, as even the slightest triggers can lead to discomfort and distress. Understanding the nuances of sensitive skin and implementing a nurturing skincare regimen is paramount for alleviating symptoms and fostering skin health.

Reactivity to External Stimuli: Sensitive skin is characterized by its heightened responsiveness to external factors. Whether it's a change in temperature, exposure to certain skincare ingredients, or environmental pollutants, sensitive skin reacts swiftly and visibly. Redness, itching, burning sensations, and stinging are common reactions, indicating the skin's vulnerability to triggers.

Redness as a Telltale Sign: A hallmark of sensitive skin, redness often manifests as an immediate response to irritation or inflammation. Whether triggered by environmental factors or skincare products, redness can be fleeting or persistent, depending on the individual's skin sensitivity and the severity of the trigger. Managing redness requires gentle care and soothing ingredients to calm inflammation and restore balance.

The Itch Factor: Itching, or pruritus, is another prevalent symptom of sensitive skin, accompanied by an irresistible urge to scratch or rub the affected area. Itching can exacerbate inflammation and redness, leading to further discomfort and potential damage to the skin barrier. Identifying and addressing the underlying cause of itching is essential for providing relief and preventing further irritation.

Avoiding Known Triggers: Individuals with sensitive skin must be vigilant about avoiding known triggers and irritants. Fragrances, harsh detergents, alcohol, and chemical preservatives are common culprits found in skincare products and household items. Opting for fragrance-free, hypoallergenic products formulated specifically for sensitive skin can help minimize the risk of adverse reactions.

Patch Testing and Gradual Introduction: When introducing new skincare products or treatments, conducting patch tests on a small area of skin is crucial for assessing compatibility and tolerance. Start with a low concentration or frequency of use, gradually increasing as tolerated. This cautious approach minimizes the risk of adverse reactions and allows the skin to acclimate to new ingredients.

Soothing Ingredients and Gentle Care: Choosing skincare products with soothing ingredients like aloe vera, chamomile, oatmeal, and ceramides can help calm inflammation and strengthen the skin barrier. Avoiding over-exfoliation and abrasive scrubs is also essential, as these can further irritate sensitive skin and exacerbate symptoms. Gentle cleansing with mild, fragrance-free products helps maintain skin health without stripping away essential moisture.

Holistic Approach to Skincare: In addition to topical skincare, adopting a holistic approach to skincare involves considering lifestyle factors that may impact sensitive skin. Practicing sun protection, managing stress levels, and maintaining a healthy diet can all contribute to overall skin health and resilience. By prioritizing gentle care, avoiding known triggers, and adopting a mindful approach to skincare, individuals with sensitive skin can achieve a calmer, healthier complexion.

2.2

Common Skin Concerns and Their Causes

Unlocking Clear, Radiant Skin
Navigating Acne and Blemish Complexities

Every woman desires a complexion that radiates health and vitality, yet the journey to achieving such skin can often be impeded by the presence of acne and blemishes. In this modern age of skincare innovations, understanding the root causes of acne breakouts remains paramount. From excess oil production to hormonal fluctuations and lifestyle habits, a multitude of factors contribute to the development of blemishes, disrupting the delicate balance of the skin and dampening one's confidence.

Excess oil production, stemming from the skin's sebaceous glands, is a common culprit behind acne breakouts. When sebum mixes with dead skin cells, it can clog pores, providing an ideal environment for acne-causing bacteria to proliferate. This excess oil production can lead to the formation of blackheads, whiteheads, and inflammatory acne lesions, compromising the skin's clarity and smoothness.

Clogged pores further exacerbate the issue, serving as breeding grounds for bacteria and contributing to the cycle of inflammation and blemishes. Through gentle exfoliation and pore-clearing treatments, individuals can unclog pores, prevent the formation of acne lesions, and promote a clearer, more radiant complexion.

The role of bacterial overgrowth, particularly Propionibacterium acnes (P. acnes), cannot be understated in the context of acne development. When trapped within clogged pores, P. acnes multiply rapidly, triggering an inflammatory response that manifests as papules, pustules, and nodules. Targeted treatments containing antibacterial agents can effectively combat bacterial overgrowth and reduce inflammation, facilitating the resolution of acne lesions.

Hormonal fluctuations, a natural part of a woman's life journey, can significantly impact sebum production and contribute to acne breakouts. Increased levels of androgens, such as testosterone, stimulate the sebaceous glands, resulting in oilier skin and a heightened risk of acne flare-ups. Hormonal acne, often characterized by deep, cystic lesions, requires specialized treatment to manage effectively and restore skin health.

Beyond biological factors, lifestyle habits play a pivotal role in acne management. Maintaining a balanced diet, managing stress levels, getting adequate sleep, and practicing sun protection are essential components of a holistic skincare regimen. By nurturing the body from within, individuals can support their skin's natural healing processes and minimize the risk of blemishes.

The path to clear, radiant skin is paved with understanding, patience, and a multifaceted approach to skincare. By addressing the root causes of acne breakouts and adopting targeted treatments and lifestyle habits, women can reclaim control over their skin and embrace their natural beauty with confidence and grace. With perseverance and dedication, the journey to unlocking clear, radiant skin is within reach for every woman.

Dryness and Dehydration
Unraveling the Causes

In the pursuit of radiant, healthy-looking skin, dryness and dehydration stand as formidable foes, casting shadows on one's complexion and dampening their confidence. Understanding the intricate web of factors that contribute to these common skin concerns is paramount for effectively addressing them and achieving optimal skin hydration. From environmental aggressors to skincare practices and genetic predispositions, let's delve into the multifaceted world of dryness and dehydration and uncover actionable insights for maintaining glowing, moisturized skin.

Environmental factors such as cold weather, low humidity, and excessive sun exposure can strip the skin of its natural moisture, leaving it feeling dry and parched. Similarly, indoor environments with central heating or air conditioning can further deplete the skin's hydration levels, creating a perfect storm for dryness and dehydration to thrive.

Our skincare routine can either nourish or compromise the skin's moisture barrier, depending on the products we use. Cleansers containing harsh ingredients like sulfates or alcohol can strip away the skin's natural oils, disrupting its delicate balance and leading to increased dryness and irritation.

While a long, hot shower may feel indulgent, it can have detrimental effects on the skin's hydration levels. Prolonged exposure to hot water can strip away the skin's natural oils, leaving it feeling dry, tight, and uncomfortable.

Maintaining adequate hydration is crucial for supporting skin health and preventing dryness and dehydration. However, factors such as inadequate water intake, excessive caffeine or alcohol consumption, and certain medications can contribute to dehydration, leaving the skin parched and lacking in moisture.

Our skincare habits can significantly impact the moisture levels of our skin. Over-exfoliation or using products with harsh ingredients can strip away the skin's protective barrier, leading to increased dryness and sensitivity. Opting for gentle, hydrating skincare products and

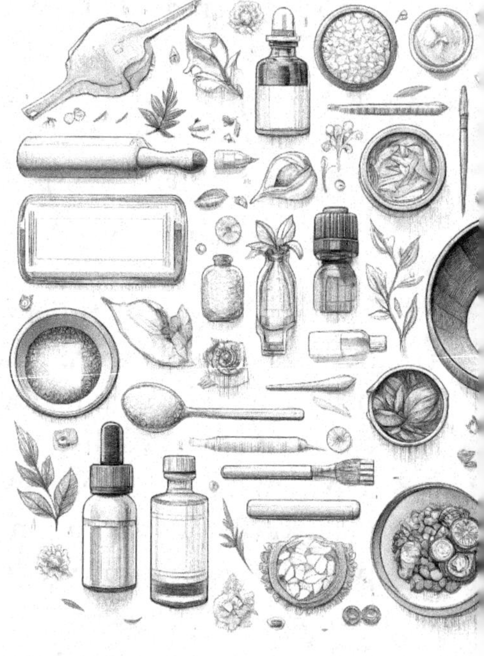

avoiding overuse of exfoliants can help maintain the skin's natural moisture balance and prevent dehydration.

Certain medical conditions, such as eczema, psoriasis, and dermatitis, can compromise the skin's barrier function, leading to increased water loss and exacerbating dryness and irritation. Seeking medical advice and treatment for these conditions can help alleviate symptoms and restore the skin's health and hydration.

As we age, the skin naturally becomes thinner and produces less oil, making it more prone to dryness and dehydration. Additionally, hormonal changes associated with menopause can further exacerbate dryness, leaving the skin feeling tight, rough, and lacking in moisture. Incorporating hydrating skincare products and practices into our routine can help support aging skin and maintain its moisture balance.

Dietary choices can also impact skin hydration, with deficiencies in essential fatty acids, vitamins, and minerals contributing to dryness and dehydration. Consuming a balanced diet rich in omega-3 fatty acids, antioxidants, and hydration-rich foods such as fruits and vegetables can help support skin health and hydration from the inside out.

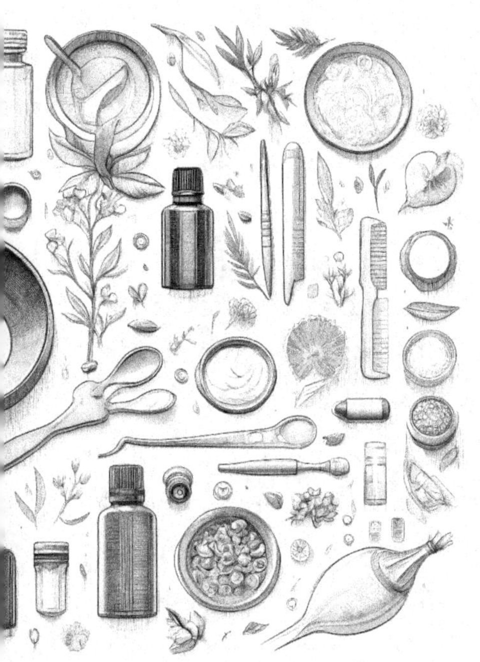

Elevated stress levels can have profound effects on skin health, increasing inflammation and disrupting the skin's barrier function. Chronic stress can lead to increased cortisol levels, which can impair the skin's ability to retain moisture and exacerbate dryness and dehydration. Incorporating stress-reducing practices such as meditation, yoga, or mindfulness can help support skin health and maintain optimal hydration levels.

Genetic factors can influence one's predisposition to dryness and dehydration, with some individuals inheriting a weaker skin barrier that is more prone to moisture loss. While we can't change our genetic makeup, understanding our skin's unique needs can help inform skincare choices and practices that support optimal hydration and overall skin health.

Addressing dryness and dehydration requires a holistic approach that takes into account various factors such as environmental influences, skincare practices, lifestyle habits, and genetic predispositions. By understanding the root causes of these common skin concerns and implementing proactive measures to support skin hydration, individuals can achieve and maintain a radiant, healthy-looking complexion for years to come.

Unlocking Dark Spots
What Makes Skin Tone Uneven?

Hyperpigmentation and uneven skin tone are common skin concerns that affect individuals of all ages and skin types. Understanding the triggers for these conditions is crucial for effectively addressing them and achieving a more balanced, radiant complexion. From sun damage to post-inflammatory hyperpigmentation (PIH) and melasma, let's explore the factors that contribute to hyperpigmentation and uneven skin tone.

Sun damage stands as one of the primary culprits behind hyperpigmentation and uneven skin tone. Prolonged exposure to ultraviolet (UV) radiation from the sun can stimulate melanin production in the skin, leading to the formation of dark spots and patches. This type of hyperpigmentation, known as solar lentigines or sun spots, often manifests on areas of the skin that receive the most sun exposure, such as the face, hands, and décolletage.

Post-inflammatory hyperpigmentation (PIH) is another common trigger for dark spots and uneven skin tone. This condition occurs because of inflammation or injury to the skin, such as acne breakouts, insect bites, or cuts. In response to the trauma, the skin produces excess melanin, resulting in the formation of dark marks or patches that linger long after the initial injury has healed.

Melasma, characterized by brown or grayish patches on the skin, is a condition that primarily affects women and is often triggered by hormonal fluctuations. Pregnancy, oral contraceptive use, and hormone replacement therapy can all contribute to the development of melasma, as can sun exposure and genetic predisposition. These dark patches typically appear on the face, particularly on the cheeks, forehead, and upper lip, and can be challenging to treat.

In addition to these primary triggers, certain lifestyle factors and skincare practices can exacerbate hyperpigmentation and uneven skin tone. Frequent sun exposure without adequate protection, such as sunscreen and protective clothing, can worsen existing pigmentation concerns and contribute to the development of new dark spots. Similarly, using harsh exfoliants or undergoing aggressive cosmetic procedures can increase skin sensitivity and trigger inflammation, leading to the formation of PIH.

Addressing hyperpigmentation and uneven skin tone requires a multifaceted approach that targets the underlying causes while promoting skin renewal and repair. Sun protection is paramount in preventing further pigmentation, with daily application of broad-spectrum sunscreen being essential, regardless of the weather or season. Additionally, incorporating ingredients such as vitamin C, niacinamide, and alpha hydroxy acids (AHAs) into your skincare routine can help fade existing dark spots and brighten the complexion over time.

For stubborn pigmentation concerns, professional treatments such as chemical peels, laser therapy, and microneedling may be recommended. These procedures work by targeting melanin-producing cells in the skin, breaking down existing pigmentation and stimulating collagen production for a more even, radiant complexion. However, it's essential to consult with a dermatologist or skincare professional before undergoing any invasive treatments to ensure they are suitable for your skin type and concerns.

Hyperpigmentation and uneven skin tone can be triggered by a variety of factors, including sun damage, post-inflammatory hyperpigmentation, and hormonal fluctuations. By understanding these triggers and adopting a comprehensive approach to skincare that includes sun protection, targeted treatments, and professional interventions when necessary, individuals can effectively address pigmentation concerns and achieve a more balanced, radiant complexion.

Why We Wrinkle
Exploring Skin Aging

As we journey through life, our skin undergoes a natural evolution, reflecting the passage of time through the appearance of wrinkles and other signs of aging. This complex process is influenced by a combination of biological factors and external forces, each playing a significant role in shaping the aging trajectory of our skin.

One of the key biological processes underlying skin aging is the gradual loss of collagen, a structural protein that provides strength and elasticity to the skin. As we age, the production of collagen slows down, leading to a decline in skin firmness and resilience.

This decrease in collagen levels contributes to the formation of wrinkles, fine lines, and sagging skin, giving rise to a more aged appearance.

In addition to intrinsic factors, external influences such as UV exposure play a pivotal role in accelerating skin aging. Chronic exposure to ultraviolet radiation from the sun damages the skin's collagen and elastin fibers, leading to premature aging signs such as wrinkles, sunspots, and uneven skin tone. Prolonged sun exposure without adequate protection can significantly expedite the aging process, making sun protection a crucial component of any anti-aging skincare regimen.

Oxidative stress is another factor that contributes to skin aging, both internally and externally. Reactive oxygen species (ROS), generated as byproducts of cellular metabolism or in response to environmental stressors, can damage DNA, proteins, and lipids in the skin, accelerating the aging process. Antioxidants play a critical role in neutralizing ROS and minimizing oxidative damage, highlighting the importance of incorporating antioxidant-rich skincare products into one's routine.

Lifestyle factors also play a significant role in shaping the aging process of the skin. Poor dietary choices, smoking, excessive alcohol consumption, and inadequate sleep can all contribute to premature skin aging. A diet rich in antioxidants, vitamins, and minerals can help support skin health and minimize oxidative stress, while avoiding smoking and excessive alcohol intake can help preserve collagen and elastin fibers in the skin.

Furthermore, stress and lack of sleep can negatively impact skin health by increasing cortisol levels and disrupting the skin's natural repair processes. Chronic stress can lead to inflammation, exacerbating skin conditions such as acne and rosacea, while insufficient sleep can impair collagen production and contribute to the formation of wrinkles and fine lines.

Genetic factors also play a role in determining how our skin ages over time. While some individuals may inherit genes that predispose them to more resilient skin, others may be more susceptible to premature aging due to genetic variations that affect collagen production, antioxidant capacity, or other factors involved in skin aging.

Environmental pollutants, such as air pollution and cigarette smoke, can also contribute to skin aging by generating free radicals and causing oxidative stress. Additionally, exposure to blue light from electronic devices has been linked to skin damage and premature aging, highlighting the importance of protecting the skin against digital pollution.

In conclusion, skin aging is a complex process influenced by a combination of biological processes and environmental factors. Collagen loss, UV exposure, oxidative stress, lifestyle choices, genetic predisposition, and environmental pollutants all contribute to the aging trajectory of our skin. By understanding these factors and adopting preventive measures such as sun protection, antioxidant supplementation, and a healthy lifestyle, we can help delay the onset of wrinkles and maintain a more youthful complexion for longer.

Sensitivity and Irritation
Finding Comfort and Confidence in Skincare

Sensitive skin and irritation pose significant challenges for many individuals, impacting their comfort and confidence in their skincare routines. Understanding the various factors that contribute to sensitivity and irritation is essential for effectively managing these concerns and maintaining skin health. From common irritants and allergens found in skincare products to environmental triggers and underlying skin conditions like eczema or rosacea, let's delve into the multifaceted world of sensitivity and irritation.

Skincare products often contain a myriad of ingredients, some of which can be potential irritants or allergens for sensitive individuals. Harsh surfactants like sulfates, fragrances, preservatives such as parabens, and certain essential oils are common culprits known to trigger sensitivity and irritation reactions. Additionally, alcohol-based products and exfoliants with abrasive particles can exacerbate skin irritation, leading to redness, itching, and discomfort.

Environmental triggers such as pollution, extreme weather conditions, and UV exposure can also contribute to skin sensitivity and irritation. Pollutants in the air can penetrate the skin barrier, causing inflammation and oxidative stress, while harsh weather conditions like cold winds or excessive heat can strip the skin of its natural oils, leading to dryness and irritation. Prolonged exposure to UV radiation from the sun can further exacerbate skin sensitivity and trigger inflammatory responses, making sun protection a crucial aspect of sensitive skin care.

Underlying skin conditions like eczema and rosacea are characterized by heightened skin sensitivity and reactivity to various triggers. Eczema, also known as atopic dermatitis, is a chronic inflammatory skin condition characterized by red, itchy rashes that can flare up in response to certain triggers such as allergens, stress, or irritants in skincare products. Similarly, rosacea is a common skin disorder characterized by facial redness, flushing, and visible blood vessels, often exacerbated by factors like sunlight, spicy foods, alcohol, and harsh skincare products.

Identifying and avoiding potential irritants and allergens in skincare products is crucial for managing sensitivity and irritation. Opting for fragrance-free, hypoallergenic formulas formulated with gentle, non-comedogenic ingredients can help minimize the risk of adverse reactions and soothe sensitive skin. Patch testing new products before full application can also help identify any potential sensitivities or allergies before they escalate into a full-blown reaction.

In addition to external factors, internal factors such as stress, hormonal fluctuations, and dietary choices can also influence skin sensitivity and reactivity. Chronic stress can weaken the skin's barrier function and increase inflammation, making it more susceptible to irritation and sensitivity reactions. Hormonal fluctuations, particularly during puberty, pregnancy, or menopause, can also impact skin health and trigger sensitivity flare-ups. Additionally, consuming inflammatory foods or allergens can exacerbate skin conditions like eczema or rosacea, further contributing to sensitivity and irritation.

Managing sensitivity and irritation requires a holistic approach that addresses both internal and external factors. Adopting a gentle skincare routine with minimalistic products formulated for sensitive skin can help reduce the risk of irritation and inflammation. Practicing stress-reducing techniques such as mindfulness, meditation, or yoga can help alleviate internal triggers and promote skin health from within. Consulting with a dermatologist or skincare professional can also provide personalized recommendations and treatment options for managing underlying skin conditions like eczema or rosacea.

Sensitivity and irritation are common concerns that can significantly impact the comfort and well-being of individuals with sensitive skin. Understanding the various triggers, including common irritants and allergens in skincare products, environmental factors, and underlying skin conditions, is essential for effectively managing these concerns and maintaining skin health. By adopting a gentle skincare routine, identifying and avoiding potential triggers, and addressing internal factors such as stress and hormonal fluctuations, individuals can achieve a calmer, more comfortable complexion.

2.3

Creating a Personalized
Skincare Routine

The Power of Cleansing
Finding the Perfect Routine for Your Skin

Cleansing is the cornerstone of any skincare routine, laying the foundation for healthy, radiant skin. Choosing the right cleanser is essential, as it can effectively remove dirt, oil, and impurities without stripping the skin's natural moisture barrier. Understanding your skin type and lifestyle is key to selecting a cleanser that meets your needs and supports your skincare goals.

For those with oily or acne-prone skin, a gel or foaming cleanser can help to effectively remove excess oil and impurities while preventing breakouts. Look for ingredients like salicylic acid or tea tree oil, known for their ability to unclog pores and reduce acne-causing bacteria. On the other hand, individuals with dry or sensitive skin may benefit from a creamy or hydrating cleanser that gently cleanses without causing irritation or dryness. Ingredients like hyaluronic acid and ceramides can help to hydrate and nourish the skin while cleansing.

In addition to considering your skin type, it's important to take your lifestyle into account when choosing a cleanser. If you wear makeup regularly or live in a city with high pollution levels, opting for a cleanser that offers thorough makeup removal and pollution protection is crucial. Micellar water or oil-based cleansers are excellent options for effectively removing makeup and impurities without stripping the skin or causing irritation.

Double cleansing has gained popularity in recent years for its ability to thoroughly cleanse the skin and improve skincare efficacy. The first step involves using an oil-based cleanser or cleansing balm to dissolve makeup, sunscreen, and excess oil on the skin's surface. This allows for a deeper cleanse in the second step, where a water-based cleanser is used to remove any remaining impurities and cleanse the skin.

Double cleansing is especially beneficial for individuals who wear heavy makeup or sunscreen, as it ensures that all traces of makeup and impurities are effectively removed from the skin. It also helps to prepare the skin for the application of skincare products, allowing active ingredients to penetrate more deeply and deliver optimal results.

In addition to choosing the right cleanser, it's important to cleanse your skin properly to maximize its benefits. Start by wetting your face with lukewarm water, then apply a small amount of cleanser to your fingertips and gently massage it into your skin using circular motions. Rinse thoroughly with water and pat your skin dry with a clean towel. Avoid using hot water, as it can strip the skin of its natural oils and cause irritation.

Consistency is key when it comes to cleansing, so aim to cleanse your skin twice daily, morning and night, to keep it clean and refreshed. However, be mindful not to over-cleanse, as this can disrupt the skin's natural moisture barrier and lead to dryness or irritation. Pay attention to how your skin responds to your cleansing routine and adjust as needed to maintain a healthy balance.

Choosing the right cleanser for your skin type and lifestyle is essential for maintaining healthy, radiant skin. Whether you have oily, dry, or sensitive skin, there is a cleanser out there to meet your needs and support your skincare goals. By understanding the importance of double cleansing for thorough makeup removal and skincare efficacy, you can achieve a clean, refreshed complexion that glows from within.

Balanced Beauty
The Essential Role of Toning

Toning is a crucial step in any skincare routine, often overlooked but essential for maintaining balanced, healthy skin. Incorporating toners or facial mists into your regimen can help balance pH levels, hydrate, and prepare the skin for subsequent skincare products. Understanding the benefits of toning and how to choose the right product for your skin type is key to unlocking its full potential.

Toners are typically water-based liquids formulated with a variety of active ingredients designed to address specific skincare concerns. One of the primary benefits of toning is restoring the skin's pH balance after cleansing. Cleansers can disrupt the skin's natural pH, which can lead to dryness, sensitivity, and other issues. Toners help to rebalance the skin's pH, creating an optimal environment for healthy skin function.

In addition to balancing pH levels, toners also serve as a hydration booster, delivering moisture to the skin and preparing it to better absorb subsequent skincare products. Hydrated skin is essential for maintaining a healthy moisture barrier, which helps protect against environmental aggressors and prevents moisture loss. Look for toners containing ingredients like hyaluronic acid, glycerin, or botanical extracts to hydrate and plump the skin.

Furthermore, toners can help to remove any remaining impurities or traces of makeup after cleansing, ensuring that the skin is thoroughly clean and ready for the application of serums, moisturizers, and treatments. This can be particularly beneficial for individuals with oily or acne-prone skin, as it helps to minimize the risk of clogged pores and breakouts.

Facial mists are another popular option for toning the skin, offering a convenient and refreshing way to hydrate and rejuvenate throughout the day. Formulated with soothing and hydrating ingredients like rose water, aloe vera, or botanical extracts, facial mists provide an instant boost of hydration and can help calm and soothe irritated or sensitive skin.

When choosing a toner or facial mist, it's essential to consider your skin type and specific skincare concerns. For oily or acne-prone skin, look for toners with ingredients like salicylic acid or witch hazel to help control oil production and minimize breakouts. Dry or sensitive skin types may benefit from hydrating toners containing gentle ingredients like chamomile or calendula to soothe and nourish the skin.

To incorporate toning into your skincare routine, simply apply a small amount of toner to a cotton pad or spritz directly onto the skin after cleansing. Gently sweep the toner across your face and neck, avoiding the delicate eye area. Allow the toner to absorb fully before applying serums, moisturizers, or treatments.

Consistency is key when it comes to toning, so aim to incorporate this step into your skincare routine morning and night for best results. With regular use, toners can help to maintain a balanced, hydrated complexion and enhance the effectiveness of your overall skincare regimen. Whether you prefer a traditional toner or a refreshing facial mist, adding this step to your routine can make a noticeable difference in the health and appearance of your skin.

Targeted Solutions
Unveiling the Power of Treatments

In the realm of skincare, treatments are the superheroes that come to the rescue when specific concerns need addressing. Serums, ampoules, and spot treatments packed with active ingredients like antioxidants, hyaluronic acid, niacinamide, or retinol are the key players in this arena. They offer targeted solutions to a myriad of skin issues, from hydration woes to fine lines and beyond. Understanding the power of these potent formulations and how to choose the right ones for your skin concerns is essential for achieving your skincare goals.

Serums are concentrated formulations designed to deliver potent ingredients deep into the skin, targeting specific concerns with precision. They come in various formulations, each tailored to address specific skincare needs. For example, antioxidant serums help protect the skin from environmental damage and premature aging, while hyaluronic acid serums provide intense hydration and plumpness. Niacinamide serums can help improve the appearance of enlarged pores, uneven skin tone, and fine lines, making them a versatile addition to any skincare routine.

Ampoules are similar to serums but are typically more concentrated and potent, offering an extra boost of targeted treatment for specific skin concerns. They often come in single-use vials or capsules, ensuring freshness and potency with each application. Ampoules are ideal for tackling stubborn skin issues like hyperpigmentation, dullness, or loss of firmness, delivering visible results in a shorter period.

Spot treatments are localized treatments designed to address specific blemishes, breakouts, or imperfections. They contain active ingredients like salicylic acid, benzoyl peroxide, or sulfur to target and treat acne lesions, reducing inflammation and promoting faster healing. Additionally, spot treatments infused with ingredients like tea tree oil or witch hazel can help soothe and calm irritated skin, making them essential for managing breakouts effectively.

When choosing treatments for your skincare routine, it's crucial to consider your skin type and specific concerns. For example, individuals with dry or dehydrated skin may benefit from hydrating serums or ampoules containing ingredients like hyaluronic acid or glycerin to replenish moisture and restore suppleness to the skin. Those with acne-prone skin may find spot treatments with salicylic acid or benzoyl peroxide effective in treating breakouts and preventing future blemishes.

Retinol is another potent ingredient commonly found in skincare treatments, known for its ability to stimulate collagen production, improve skin texture, and reduce the appearance of fine lines and wrinkles. However, it can also cause irritation, especially for those with sensitive or reactive skin. When incorporating retinol into your skincare routine, start with a lower concentration and gradually increase frequency to minimize the risk of irritation.

To incorporate treatments into your skincare routine, apply them after cleansing and toning, but before moisturizing. Gently massage a few drops of serum or ampoule onto your face and neck, focusing on areas of concern. For spot treatments, apply a small amount directly onto blemishes or imperfections and allow it to absorb fully before applying other products.

Consistency is key when it comes to treatments, so aim to use them regularly as part of your skincare routine to achieve optimal results. With the right combination of serums, ampoules, and spot treatments, you can effectively target specific concerns and achieve a healthier, more radiant complexion.

Moisturizing 101
The Essential Step for Happy Skin

Moisturizing is the unsung hero of skincare, playing a pivotal role in maintaining skin health and vitality. Whether your skin is dry, oily, or somewhere in between, finding the right moisturizer is key to keeping it hydrated, nourished, and balanced. From lightweight lotions to rich creams and nourishing oils, there's a moisturizer out there to suit every skin type and climate. Understanding the importance of moisturizing and how to choose the right product for your skin's needs is essential for achieving a healthy, radiant complexion.

Hydrating the skin is essential for maintaining its moisture balance and preventing dryness, flakiness, and irritation. Moisturizers work by creating a protective barrier on the skin's surface, locking in moisture and preventing water loss throughout the day. They also help to replenish the skin's natural lipid barrier, which can become compromised due to environmental stressors, harsh cleansers, or aging.

Nourishing the skin with moisturizers is equally important for supporting its overall health and function. Moisturizers contain ingredients like humectants, emollients, and occlusives, which work together to hydrate, soften, and soothe the skin. Humectants like hyaluronic acid and glycerin attract moisture from the environment and bind it to the skin, keeping it hydrated and plump. Emollients like ceramides and squalane help to smooth and soften the skin's surface, while occlusives like petrolatum and shea butter seal in moisture and prevent dehydration.

Choosing the right moisturizer for your skin type is crucial for ensuring optimal results. For dry or dehydrated skin, opt for rich, creamy moisturizers that provide intense hydration and nourishment. Look for ingredients like ceramides, fatty acids, and natural oils like jojoba or avocado oil to replenish moisture and restore suppleness to the skin. Individuals with oily or acne-prone skin should opt for lightweight, oil-free moisturizers that hydrate without clogging pores or exacerbating breakouts. Gel-based or water-based formulas are ideal for oily skin types, providing hydration without adding excess oiliness.

Consider your climate when choosing a moisturizer, as the environment can impact your skin's hydration needs. In dry or cold climates, opt for heavier, more emollient moisturizers to provide extra protection against moisture loss. In humid climates, lightweight, oil-free moisturizers are preferable to prevent excess oiliness and congestion.

In addition to choosing the right moisturizer, it's essential to apply it correctly to maximize its benefits. After cleansing and toning, apply a small amount of moisturizer to your face and neck, using gentle, upward strokes to massage it into the skin. Allow the moisturizer to absorb fully before applying sunscreen or makeup.

Consistency is key when it comes to moisturizing, so aim to apply moisturizer twice daily, morning and night, to keep your skin hydrated and nourished. Pay attention to how your skin responds to different moisturizers and adjust your routine as needed to achieve the best results. With the right moisturizer and a consistent skincare routine, you can maintain a healthy, radiant complexion year-round.

Sun Protection
Prioritizing Daily Defense

In the domain of skincare, few measures are as paramount as sun protection. The sun's rays, while a source of warmth and vitality, can wreak havoc on our skin when left unshielded. From premature aging to hyperpigmentation and even the risk of skin cancer, the consequences of unprotected sun exposure are manifold. Therefore, in our pursuit of healthy, radiant skin, prioritizing daily sun protection with broad-spectrum SPF products is non-negotiable.

Sunscreen, often hailed as the cornerstone of sun protection, acts as a shield against the harmful effects of ultraviolet (UV) radiation. Broad-spectrum sunscreens, in particular, offer protection against both UVA and UVB rays, safeguarding the skin against a broad spectrum of damage. UVA rays penetrate deep into the skin, causing premature aging and contributing to the development of skin cancer, while UVB rays primarily affect the skin's outer layers, leading to sunburn and skin cancer.

By incorporating broad-spectrum SPF products into our daily skincare routine, we fortify our skin's natural defenses against these harmful rays. This proactive approach not only helps prevent visible signs of aging, such as fine lines, wrinkles, and age spots, but also mitigates the risk of more serious conditions, including melanoma and other forms of skin cancer.

Furthermore, consistent sun protection is imperative for maintaining an even complexion and preventing hyperpigmentation. UV exposure can trigger the overproduction of melanin, resulting in dark spots, uneven skin tone, and melasma. By applying sunscreen diligently, we shield our skin from these pigmentary changes, preserving its clarity and luminosity.

In our modern-day lifestyles, where outdoor activities, commuting, and even incidental sun exposure are commonplace, the need for sun protection extends beyond recreational sunbathing. Incorporating broad-spectrum SPF products into our daily skincare regimen is a proactive measure—one that transcends seasons and climates.

When selecting a sunscreen, opt for formulations that offer broad-spectrum protection with an SPF of 30 or higher, as recommended by dermatologists. Additionally, choose products that suit your skin type and preferences, whether you prefer lightweight lotions, hydrating creams, or tinted formulations for added coverage.

Prioritizing daily sun protection with broad-spectrum SPF products is a fundamental aspect of maintaining healthy, radiant skin. By integrating this simple yet crucial step into our skincare routine, we empower ourselves to not only preserve our skin's youthfulness and vitality but also safeguard our long-term skin health.

Chapter 3

Essential Ingredients for DIY Skincare

Forget store-bought concoctions shrouded in mystery. This chapter equips you with the arsenal you need to become a DIY natural skincare alchemist. We're talking potent botanical extracts, nourishing carrier oils, and the power to craft personalized formulas that leave your skin singing.

Here's the deal: understanding the properties and benefits of these natural powerhouses unlocks a treasure trove of possibilities. We'll delve into the world of carrier oils like jojoba and grapeseed, exploring their hydrating prowess. Botanical extracts like green tea and calendula become your allies in soothing irritation and combating signs of aging.

Imagine whipping up a gentle cleanser infused with calming chamomile for a touch of serenity. Or, perhaps a luxurious moisturizer enriched with the age-defying properties of rosehip oil is more your style? See where we're going? The possibilities are as endless as your creativity.

This chapter isn't just about filling your shelves with fancy bottles; it's about empowerment. By mastering the language of natural ingredients, you'll gain the confidence to curate a skincare routine that celebrates the unique needs of your skin. So, grab your metaphorical mortar and pestle, and let's unlock the magic of nature's apothecary, one potent ingredient at a time.

3.1

The Power of Plants: Essential Oils and Extracts

Harnessing Nature's Power
The Wonders of Essential Oils in DIY Skincare

Essential oils have been prized for centuries for their aromatic essences and potent therapeutic properties. Derived from various parts of plants through methods like steam distillation or cold pressing, these concentrated botanical extracts offer a myriad of benefits for skincare. From their anti-inflammatory and antibacterial properties to their soothing and calming effects, essential oils are versatile ingredients that can elevate your DIY skincare routine to new heights.

One of the most remarkable aspects of essential oils is their ability to address a wide range of skincare concerns, thanks to their diverse chemical compositions. For example, tea tree oil, extracted from the leaves of the Melaleuca alternifolia tree, is renowned for its potent antibacterial and antimicrobial properties, making it a popular choice for treating acne and blemishes. Lavender oil, on the other hand, is prized for its calming and soothing effects, making it ideal for sensitive or irritated skin.

The process of extracting essential oils from plants is as fascinating as the oils themselves. Steam distillation is one of the most common methods used to extract essential oils from aromatic plants. In this process, steam is passed through the plant material, causing the essential oils to evaporate and then condense into a liquid form. Cold pressing, on the other hand, is used to extract essential oils from citrus fruits like lemon or orange. In this method, the rinds of the fruits are mechanically pressed to release the oils.

When incorporating essential oils into DIY skincare recipes, it's essential to choose high-quality, pure oils to ensure maximum efficacy and safety. Look for oils that are labeled as 100% pure and therapeutic grade, and avoid synthetic fragrances or adulterated oils that may contain harmful chemicals or additives. Additionally, always perform a patch test before using any essential oil topically to check for sensitivity or allergic reactions.

Some essential oils are known for their anti-inflammatory properties, making them excellent choices for soothing irritated or inflamed skin conditions like eczema or rosacea. Chamomile oil, for example, contains compounds that help reduce redness and inflammation, making it a gentle and effective option for sensitive skin types. Similarly, rose oil has anti-inflammatory properties that can help calm and soothe irritated skin while promoting healing and regeneration.

In addition to their therapeutic benefits for the skin, essential oils also offer aromatic benefits that can enhance your overall well-being. The aroma of essential oils can positively impact mood and emotions, promoting relaxation, stress relief, and mental clarity. Diffusing essential oils or incorporating them into skincare products can create a spa-like experience at home, providing a moment of self-care and rejuvenation.

When using essential oils in DIY skincare, it's essential to dilute them properly to avoid skin irritation or sensitization. Carrier oils like jojoba oil, sweet almond oil, or coconut oil are commonly used to dilute essential oils and create safe and effective skincare formulations. The general rule of thumb is to use no more than 1-2% essential oil concentration in your skincare recipes to ensure safety and efficacy.

Experimenting with essential oils in DIY skincare can be a rewarding and empowering experience, allowing you to customize your skincare products to suit your unique needs and preferences. Whether you're looking to address specific skin concerns or simply indulge in the aromatic delights of nature, essential oils offer a world of possibilities for enhancing your skincare routine. With a little knowledge and creativity, you can harness the power of these aromatic essences to nourish, heal, and beautify your skin naturally.

Nature's Bounty
The Marvels of Botanical Extracts

Botanical extracts are nature's gift to skincare, offering a treasure trove of vitamins, antioxidants, and phytochemicals that nourish, protect, and rejuvenate the skin. Extracted from various parts of plants through meticulous processes, these potent ingredients have long been prized for their ability to enhance skin health and beauty. From green tea extract and chamomile extract to calendula extract and beyond, let's explore the wonders of botanical extracts and their transformative effects on the skin.

Green tea extract is a powerhouse ingredient packed with antioxidants like catechins and polyphenols, which help neutralize free radicals and protect the skin from environmental damage. It also has anti-inflammatory properties that can soothe and calm irritated skin, making it ideal for sensitive or acne-prone skin types. Additionally, green tea extract contains caffeine, which can help reduce puffiness and tighten the skin, making it a popular choice for eye creams and serums.

Chamomile extract is renowned for its calming and soothing properties, making it a beloved ingredient in skincare products designed for sensitive or reactive skin. It contains chamazulene, a compound that has anti-inflammatory effects and can help reduce redness and irritation. Chamomile extract also has antioxidant properties that help protect the skin from oxidative stress and premature aging, making it a valuable addition to anti-aging skincare formulations.

Calendula extract, derived from the marigold flower, is prized for its healing and anti-inflammatory properties. It contains compounds like flavonoids and triterpenoids, which promote skin regeneration and wound healing. Calendula extract is often used to soothe and alleviate various skin conditions, including eczema, psoriasis, and dermatitis. Its gentle yet effective nature makes it suitable for all skin types, including sensitive or inflamed skin.

When incorporating botanical extracts into skincare formulations, it's essential to choose high-quality extracts that are extracted using gentle methods to preserve their potency and efficacy. Cold pressing and CO_2 extraction are two common methods used to extract botanical extracts without exposing them to heat or harsh chemicals, ensuring that their beneficial properties remain intact.

Botanical extracts can be found in a wide range of skincare products, including cleansers, toners, serums, moisturizers, and masks. They are often included for their specific skincare benefits, such as brightening, hydrating, soothing, or anti-aging effects. When selecting skincare products containing botanical extracts, it's essential to consider your skin type and specific concerns to ensure compatibility and effectiveness.

In addition to their skincare benefits, botanical extracts also offer aromatic delights that can enhance your overall sensory experience. The natural fragrances of plants like chamomile, lavender, and rose can evoke feelings of calmness and relaxation, making skincare rituals a luxurious and indulgent experience.

Whether you're seeking to address specific skin concerns or simply pamper yourself with the goodness of nature, botanical extracts offer a holistic approach to skincare that nourishes both the skin and the soul. With their potent blend of vitamins, antioxidants, and phytochemicals, these natural wonders have the power to transform your skincare routine and unveil a radiant, glowing complexion.

3.2

Nutrient-Rich Oils and Butters for Nourished Skin

Nourishing Foundations
Harnessing the Power of Carrier Oils

Carrier oils, often referred to as base oils, are the unsung heroes of skincare, providing a nourishing and protective base for essential oils and other active ingredients. Derived from seeds, nuts, and fruits, these versatile oils boast a diverse array of fatty acids, vitamins, and antioxidants that offer a multitude of benefits for the skin. From jojoba oil and rosehip seed oil to argan oil and beyond, let's explore the wonders of carrier oils and their unique contributions to skincare.

Jojoba oil, derived from the seeds of the jojoba plant, is prized for its remarkable similarity to the skin's natural sebum. Rich in vitamins E and B-complex, as well as essential fatty acids, jojoba oil is easily absorbed by the skin, making it an excellent moisturizer for all skin types. Its balancing and non-comedogenic properties make it particularly beneficial for oily or acne-prone skin, helping to regulate sebum production and prevent breakouts.

Rosehip seed oil, extracted from the seeds of the wild rose plant, is revered for its potent anti-aging properties. Packed with vitamins A, C, and E, as well as essential fatty acids like omega-3 and omega-6, rosehip seed oil promotes cell regeneration, boosts collagen production, and reduces the appearance of fine lines and wrinkles. Its lightweight texture and fast absorption rate make it suitable for all skin types, including dry, mature, or sensitive skin.

Argan oil, often referred to as "liquid gold," is extracted from the kernels of the argan tree native to Morocco. Rich in antioxidants, vitamin E, and essential fatty acids like oleic and linoleic acid, argan oil nourishes and moisturizes the skin while providing protection against environmental stressors. Its rejuvenating properties make it an excellent choice for addressing signs of aging, such as dryness, dullness, and loss of elasticity.

When choosing carrier oils for skincare, it's essential to consider their unique fatty acid compositions, absorption rates, and skin benefits. For example, oils high in linoleic acid, such as **grapeseed oil** and **hemp seed oil**, are lightweight and fast-absorbing, making them ideal for oily or acne-prone skin. In contrast, oils high in oleic acid, such as **sweet almond oil** and **avocado oil**, are richer and more nourishing, making them suitable for dry or mature skin types.

In addition to their moisturizing properties, carrier oils also serve as excellent vehicles for delivering essential oils and other active ingredients deeper into the skin. When combined with essential oils, carrier oils help dilute the potent essences and reduce the risk of skin irritation or sensitization. They also help to enhance the absorption and efficacy of essential oils, allowing them to penetrate the skin more effectively and deliver their therapeutic benefits.

Incorporating carrier oils into your skincare routine is simple and versatile. They can be used alone as moisturizers, massage oils, or makeup removers, or blended with essential oils and other botanical extracts to create customized skincare formulations tailored to your skin's specific needs. Whether you're looking to hydrate, nourish, or rejuvenate your skin, carrier oils offer a natural and effective solution for achieving a healthy, radiant complexion.

Carrier oils are indispensable allies in the quest for beautiful, healthy skin. With their diverse array of fatty acids, vitamins, and antioxidants, oils like jojoba, rosehip seed, and argan oil offer a wealth of benefits for all skin types. By understanding their unique properties and incorporating them into your skincare routine, you can unlock the transformative power of nature and unveil a complexion that radiates health and vitality.

Luxurious Treasures
The Transformative Power of Plant Butters

Plant butters are nature's luxurious treasures, prized for their rich texture, emollient properties, and ability to deeply nourish and protect the skin. Derived from the kernels or seeds of various plants, these decadent butters offer a wealth of benefits for skincare, particularly for those with dry, dehydrated, or mature skin types. From shea butter and cocoa butter to mango butter and beyond, let's embark on a journey to discover the wonders of plant butters and their transformative effects on the skin.

Shea butter, derived from the nuts of the shea tree native to Africa, is celebrated for its exceptional moisturizing and emollient properties. Rich in fatty acids, vitamins, and antioxidants, shea butter forms a protective barrier on the skin's surface, locking in moisture and preventing dehydration. Its creamy texture and gentle nature make it suitable for all skin types, from dry and sensitive to normal and combination. Shea butter is also known for its soothing and anti-inflammatory properties, making it an excellent choice for calming irritated or inflamed skin.

Cocoa butter, extracted from the beans of the cacao tree, is renowned for its rich, chocolatey aroma and velvety texture. Packed with fatty acids, antioxidants, and phytochemicals, cocoa butter deeply moisturizes and softens the skin, leaving it smooth, supple, and glowing. Its high concentration of oleic acid and stearic acid provides long-lasting hydration and helps improve skin elasticity, making it an ideal choice for preventing and reducing the appearance of stretch marks and scars.

Mango butter, derived from the kernels of the mango fruit, is a luxurious butter known for its lightweight texture and non-greasy feel. Rich in vitamins A, C, and E, as well as essential fatty acids, mango butter nourishes and revitalizes the skin, leaving it soft, plump, and radiant. Its antioxidant properties help protect the skin from environmental damage and premature aging, while its emollient nature seals in moisture and prevents moisture loss. Mango butter is particularly beneficial for dry, mature, or sun-damaged skin, providing intense hydration and rejuvenation.

When incorporating plant butters into skincare formulations, it's essential to choose high-quality, unrefined butters to ensure maximum efficacy and purity. Unrefined butters retain their natural color, aroma, and nutrient content, making them more potent and beneficial for the skin. Look for butters that are cold-pressed or minimally processed to preserve their beneficial properties and avoid refined or bleached butters that may contain additives or contaminants.

Plant butters can be used in a variety of skincare products, including creams, lotions, balms, and body butters. They can be applied directly to the skin as a moisturizer or incorporated into DIY skincare recipes to enhance their nourishing and hydrating properties. Whether used alone or in combination with other botanical ingredients, plant butters offer a luxurious and effective solution for achieving soft, smooth, and radiant skin.

Plant butters are nature's gifts to skincare, offering a wealth of benefits for dry, dehydrated, or mature skin. From shea butter and cocoa butter to mango butter and beyond, these luxurious butters deeply moisturize, soften, and protect the skin, leaving it healthy, radiant, and rejuvenated. By incorporating plant butters into your skincare routine, you can indulge in the pampering and nourishing goodness of nature and unveil a complexion that glows with vitality and beauty.

3.3

Natural Additives
for Customized Formulations

Invaluable Additions
The Beauty Secrets of Clays and Powders

Clays and powders are potent ingredients that have been cherished for centuries for their remarkable skincare benefits. From detoxifying and exfoliating to clarifying and soothing, these natural wonders offer a multitude of advantages for achieving healthy, radiant skin. Let's delve into the transformative properties of mineral-rich clays like kaolin, bentonite, and French green clay, as well as powdered botanicals such as oatmeal, rice flour, and spirulina, and discover how they can elevate your skincare routine to new heights.

Kaolin clay, also known as white clay, is a gentle yet effective option for all skin types, including sensitive and dry skin. Rich in minerals such as silica, magnesium, and calcium, kaolin clay works to absorb excess oil, unclog pores, and detoxify the skin without stripping away its natural moisture. Its mild exfoliating properties help to remove dead skin cells, leaving the skin feeling soft, smooth, and refreshed. Kaolin clay is particularly beneficial for those with acne-prone skin, as it helps to reduce inflammation and prevent breakouts.

Bentonite clay, derived from volcanic ash, is renowned for its powerful detoxifying properties. Due to its high absorption capacity, bentonite clay draws out impurities, toxins, and excess oil from the skin, making it an excellent choice for deep cleansing and purifying. Its alkaline pH helps to balance the skin's acidity, reducing inflammation and promoting healing. Bentonite clay is ideal for oily and acne-prone skin types, as well as those with congested pores or blemishes.

French green clay, also known as sea clay or montmorillonite clay, is prized for its mineral-rich composition and vibrant green color. Rich in magnesium, calcium, potassium, and other trace minerals, French green clay helps to stimulate circulation, tighten pores, and improve skin tone and texture. Its absorbent properties make it effective at removing impurities, excess oil, and toxins from the skin, leaving it clarified and revitalized. French green clay is suitable for all skin types, particularly combination and oily skin, as it helps to balance oil production and control shine.

In addition to clays, powdered botanicals offer gentle exfoliation and soothing effects for the skin. **Oatmeal**, for example, is a natural exfoliant and anti-inflammatory ingredient that helps to calm irritation, relieve itching, and promote healing. Its gentle abrasive texture sloughs away dead skin cells, revealing a smoother, more radiant complexion. Oatmeal is suitable for all skin types, including sensitive and eczema-prone skin, as it provides nourishment and hydration without causing irritation.

Rice flour, derived from finely milled rice grains, is another excellent option for gentle exfoliation and brightening. Rich in vitamins, minerals, and amino acids, rice flour helps to remove dead skin cells, improve skin texture, and fade dark spots and hyperpigmentation. Its fine texture makes it suitable for all skin types, including sensitive skin, as it provides gentle yet effective exfoliation without causing irritation.

Spirulina, a nutrient-rich algae powder, offers a host of benefits for the skin, including detoxification, hydration, and nourishment. Packed with vitamins, minerals, antioxidants, and amino acids, spirulina helps to purify and revitalize the skin, leaving it glowing with health and vitality. Its soothing and anti-inflammatory properties make it particularly beneficial for sensitive or acne-prone skin, as it helps to calm redness, reduce inflammation, and promote healing.

Incorporating clays and powders into your skincare routine is simple and versatile. They can be used alone as masks or cleansers or combined with other ingredients to create customized skincare formulations tailored to your skin's specific needs. Whether you're looking to detoxify, exfoliate, or soothe your skin, clays and powders offer natural and effective solutions for achieving a healthy, radiant complexion.

Clays and powders are invaluable additions to any skincare arsenal, offering a wealth of benefits for detoxifying, exfoliating, and clarifying the skin. From mineral-rich clays like kaolin, bentonite, and French green clay to powdered botanicals such as oatmeal, rice flour, and spirulina, these natural wonders provide gentle yet effective solutions for achieving a radiant, healthy complexion. By harnessing the power of nature's treasures, you can unveil the beauty of your skin and embrace a renewed sense of confidence and vitality.

Hydration Heroes
Harnessing the Power of Humectants

Ever craved that dewy, plump complexion that seems to radiate health? The secret lies in understanding your skin's natural moisture levels and how to support them. Enter humectants and hydrators, the heroes of a naturally hydrated and healthy glow.

These moisture-attracting compounds, including glycerin, hyaluronic acid, and honey, possess a remarkable ability to draw moisture from the environment and bind it to the skin, promoting hydration, suppleness, and a coveted plumpness.

Humectants function as the unsung heroes of hydration, working tirelessly to replenish the skin's moisture reserves and restore its natural balance. **Glycerin**, a stalwart in skincare formulations, forms a protective barrier on the skin's surface, locking in moisture and preventing dehydration. Its humectant properties not only hydrate the skin but also impart a soft, smooth texture, ensuring a radiant complexion.

Similarly, **hyaluronic acid** stands out as a veritable hydration powerhouse, capable of holding up to 1000 times its weight in water. This potent humectant penetrates deep into the skin, delivering intense hydration and plumping fine lines and wrinkles from within. By infusing the skin with moisture, hyaluronic acid restores elasticity, resilience, and a youthful glow.

Nature's bounty also offers an array of humectant-rich treasures, with **honey** emerging as a beloved hydrating ingredient. Renowned for its nourishing properties, honey attracts moisture to the skin while providing essential nutrients and antioxidants. As a natural humectant, honey soothes, softens, and revitalizes the skin, unveiling a luminous complexion that radiates health and vitality.

Incorporating humectants into your DIY skincare formulations is a surefire way to elevate their hydrating potential and unlock the secrets to plump, luminous skin. Whether crafting moisturizers, serums, or masks, harnessing the power of glycerin, hyaluronic acid, and honey ensures that your creations deliver unparalleled moisture retention and skin-quenching benefits.

To maximize the efficacy of humectants in your skincare routine, it's essential to pair them with occlusive agents that lock in moisture and prevent transepidermal water loss. Emollients such as plant oils and butters provide a protective barrier, sealing in hydration and enhancing the overall effectiveness of humectants.

Safeguarding Skincare
The Role of Preservatives and Antioxidants

Preservatives and antioxidants play crucial roles in the formulation of skincare products, ensuring their stability, efficacy, and longevity. In the domain of homemade skincare, natural alternatives such as vitamin E oil, grapefruit seed extract, and rosemary extract serve as effective preservatives, while ingredients like vitamin C, green tea extract, and rosehip oil provide potent antioxidant benefits. Let's explore how these essential components safeguard skincare formulations and promote skin health and vitality.

Natural preservatives are essential for preventing microbial growth and spoilage in homemade skincare products, extending their shelf life and maintaining their efficacy over time. **Vitamin E oil**, derived from tocopherols, is a popular choice for its antioxidant properties and ability to inhibit oxidation, thereby preserving the freshness of oils and preventing rancidity. It also helps to protect the skin from environmental stressors and free radical damage, promoting overall skin health and vitality.

Grapefruit seed extract is another effective natural preservative known for its antimicrobial and antifungal properties. Rich in polyphenols and flavonoids, grapefruit seed extract helps to inhibit the growth of bacteria, yeast, and mold, ensuring the safety and stability of skincare formulations. It is particularly useful in water-based products like toners and lotions, where microbial contamination is more likely to occur.

Rosemary extract is prized for its potent antioxidant and antimicrobial properties, making it an excellent choice for preserving homemade skincare products. Its high content of rosmarinic acid and carnosic acid helps to neutralize free radicals, protect against oxidative stress, and extend the shelf life of formulations. Rosemary extract also offers soothing and anti-inflammatory benefits for the skin, making it a versatile ingredient in skincare formulations.

Antioxidants play a critical role in protecting the skin from oxidative damage caused by environmental stressors, UV radiation, and pollution, which can lead to premature aging, inflammation, and skin disorders. **Vitamin C**, a powerful antioxidant, helps to neutralize free radicals, stimulate collagen production, and brighten the complexion, promoting a youthful, radiant appearance. Incorporating vitamin C into skincare formulations can help to improve skin texture, reduce hyperpigmentation, and enhance overall skin health.

Green tea extract is rich in polyphenols, catechins, and epigallo-catechin gallate (EGCG), potent antioxidants that help to protect the skin from UV damage, reduce inflammation, and prevent collagen degradation. Studies have shown that green tea extract can help to improve skin tone, texture, and elasticity, making it an excellent ingredient for anti-aging and sun protection formulations. It also offers soothing and anti-inflammatory benefits for sensitive or irritated skin, making it suitable for a wide range of skin types.

Rosehip oil is prized for its high concentration of vitamins A, C, and E, as well as essential fatty acids, antioxidants, and phyto-chemicals. It helps to repair and regenerate the skin, improve elasticity, and fade scars, hyperpigmentation, and fine lines. Its antioxidant properties help to protect the skin from oxidative stress and free radical damage, promoting a healthy, youthful complexion.

Incorporating natural preservatives and antioxidants into homemade skincare formulations is essential for ensuring their stability, efficacy, and safety. By harnessing the power of ingredients like vitamin E oil, grapefruit seed extract, rosemary extract, vitamin C, green tea extract, and rosehip oil, individuals can create skincare products that not only nourish and protect the skin but also promote long-term skin health and vitality. With these essential components, homemade skincare becomes a potent tool for achieving radiant, youthful-looking skin.By familiarizing yourself with these essential skincare ingredients, you'll be equipped to formulate a wide range of DIY natural skincare products, from cleansers and moisturizers to serums and masks, tailored to your skin's unique needs and preferences.

Chapter 4

Tools of the Trade:
Equip Yourself for Success

The creation of your dedicated workspace becomes a significant first step. This haven, a sanctuary for both creativity and meticulous formulation, will witness the transformation of nature's bounty into personalized elixirs designed to nourish your unique skin. But before the magic begins, we must address the importance of assembling your essential tools – the instruments that will facilitate smooth, efficient creation and, most importantly, ensure the safety and hygiene of your products.

Accuracy forms the cornerstone of successful DIY skincare. Imagine a delicate symphony composed of various ingredients, each playing a vital role in the final composition. Here, your measuring tools become the conductor's baton, ensuring each note hits the perfect pitch. A well-equipped set of graduated measuring spoons and cups, along with a kitchen scale for those precise moments, becomes paramount. Inaccurate measurements can disrupt the delicate balance of your formulations, potentially rendering them ineffective or even irritating to your skin.

Hygiene is another crucial aspect to consider within your haven. Imagine crafting a luxurious moisturizer, only to have it become a breeding ground for unwanted bacteria. To prevent such a scenario, a selection of heat-resistant glass beakers and Pyrex measuring cups become your sterilizing allies. By gently simmering them in water, you create a clean and sanitized environment for your ingredients to mingle. Stainless steel bowls and spatulas join the ensemble, offering non-reactive and easily cleaned surfaces for mixing your creations.

While precision and hygiene are paramount, let us not forget the joy of creative expression. A whisk, reminiscent of a conductor's baton in a different light, can help you whip up luxurious body butters. An immersion blender, with its gentle yet powerful emulsification capabilities, becomes your secret weapon for crafting silky smooth lotions and creams.

The tools you assemble aren't merely physical objects; they become an extension of your commitment to precision, hygiene, and of course, creativity. With the right equipment and knowledge at your fingertips, you'll be well on your way to crafting personalized skincare solutions that not only nourish your skin but also celebrate the joy of DIY discovery within your dedicated haven.

4.1

Essential Equipment
for Skincare Crafting

Mixing Bowls
Indispensable Tools for DIY Skincare Formulation

Mixing bowls serve as indispensable tools in the realm of DIY skincare formulation, offering a foundation for blending ingredients and crafting personalized products tailored to individual skin needs. These humble vessels play a crucial role in the skincare creation process, providing a platform for experimentation, innovation, and creativity. In this essay, we'll explore the significance of mixing bowls in DIY skincare and delve into key considerations for selecting the optimal bowls for your formulations.

First and foremost, mixing bowls facilitate the blending of various skincare ingredients, allowing artisans to combine oils, butters, botanical extracts, and other components to create unique formulations. Whether crafting nourishing creams, revitalizing masks, or exfoliating scrubs, mixing bowls provide a central space for amalgamating ingredients and achieving homogeneity in skincare products.

The size variability of mixing bowls is essential for accommodating different batch sizes and formulation needs. Smaller bowls are suitable for precise measurements and small-scale experiments, while larger bowls cater to bulk production and facilitate efficient mixing of larger quantities. This versatility enables skincare enthusiasts to adapt their formulations to specific requirements and production scales.

When selecting mixing bowls, the choice of materials is paramount to ensure the safety and efficacy of skincare creations. Non-reactive materials such as stainless steel, glass, or ceramic are preferred, as they do not interact with skincare ingredients and maintain the integrity of formulations. These materials also facilitate easy cleaning and sanitization, crucial for maintaining hygiene standards in skincare preparation.

Heat resistance is another important consideration, particularly when working with heat-sensitive ingredients or processes such as melting oils or heating water baths. Opting for mixing bowls that can withstand high temperatures ensures safe and efficient handling of ingredients without compromising product quality or safety.

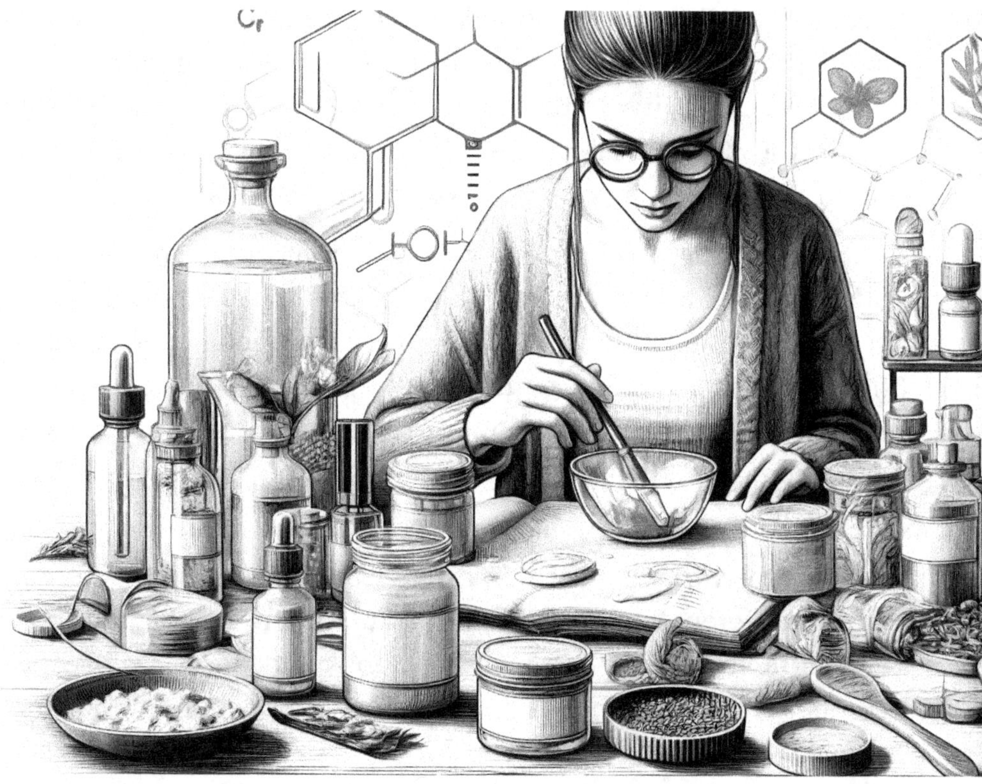

Stability and durability are fundamental attributes of mixing bowls, as they prevent spills, accidents, or disruptions during the formulation process. Bowls with sturdy bases, non-slip bottoms, or ergonomic designs offer stability on various surfaces and minimize the risk of mishaps, providing peace of mind to DIY skincare artisans.

Transparency is a beneficial feature in mixing bowls, allowing artisans to monitor the blending process and assess the consistency, texture, and color of formulations. Transparent or translucent bowls provide visibility of ingredients, enabling precise measurements and ensuring thorough mixing for uniform skincare products.

Multipurpose functionality enhances the utility of mixing bowls, with features such as lids for convenient storage, pouring spouts for easy transfer of mixtures, or nesting designs for space-saving storage. These additional attributes streamline the skincare formulation process and enhance user experience, making DIY skincare more accessible and enjoyable.

Environmental considerations are increasingly important in the selection of mixing bowls, with a growing emphasis on sustainability and eco-conscious practices. Opting for reusable materials like glass or stainless steel reduces waste and minimizes environmental impact, aligning with the principles of sustainable skincare formulation.

Budget-friendly options are also available, catering to DIY enthusiasts with varying financial constraints. Sets of mixing bowls or multipurpose designs offer affordability without compromising quality, enabling aspiring artisans to embark on their skincare formulation journey without breaking the bank.

Personal preference plays a significant role in the selection of mixing bowls, with artisans choosing bowls that complement their skincare formulation process and aesthetic preferences. Factors such as design, ergonomics, and aesthetics influence the choice of bowls, allowing individuals to express their creativity and style in DIY skincare endeavors.

Measure Up
The Indispensable Role of Precision Tools

In DIY skincare, precision is the secret ingredient that separates mediocrity from mastery. Measuring tools, from spoons and cups to scales, are the unsung heroes that ensure every concoction is crafted with accuracy and care. These tools are not just utensils; they are the guiding compass that leads skincare enthusiasts on a journey to formulation excellence.

Measuring spoons, the small but mighty players in the toolkit, provide precise increments for delicate ingredients. Whether it's a pinch of botanical extract or a drop of essential oil, these spoons ensure that every addition is measured to perfection, maintaining the integrity and potency of the formulation.

Meanwhile, measuring cups offer a versatile solution for larger volumes of liquids and powders. With clear markings and various capacities, they provide the flexibility needed to measure oils, water-based ingredients, and powdered substances accurately, streamlining the formulation process.

For those seeking the utmost accuracy, digital scales are indispensable companions. These precision instruments leave no room for guesswork, delivering exact measurements in grams or ounces. With scales, skincare artisans can achieve meticulous control over ingredient quantities, ensuring consistency across batches.

Consistency is the cornerstone of effective skincare formulations. By using precise measurements, artisans can replicate their recipes with confidence, knowing that each batch will yield the same exceptional results. This reliability builds trust with customers and sets a standard of excellence in the world of DIY skincare.

Beyond consistency, accurate measurements also promote safety in skincare formulations. Overdosing or underdosing potent ingredients can lead to adverse reactions or compromised efficacy. Measuring tools provide the guardrails that keep formulations within safe and effective ranges, protecting both the user and the product.

Moreover, these tools enhance efficiency by minimizing guesswork and streamlining the formulation process. Instead of wasting time on imprecise measurements, artisans can focus their energy on creativity and innovation, exploring new ingredients and experimenting with novel formulations.

Investing in high-quality measuring tools is a testament to a commitment to excellence. Just as a painter invests in quality brushes to create masterpieces, skincare enthusiasts prioritize precision to craft products that deliver exceptional results and exceed expectations.

Whip It Good
The Power of Handheld Immersion Blenders

Achieving the perfect texture and consistency is often a balancing act. Enter the handheld immersion blender, a versatile tool that serves as the secret weapon in creating smooth and stable formulations like creams and lotions. With its ability to emulsify oil and water-based ingredients seamlessly, this handheld marvel elevates skincare crafting to new heights.

Unlike traditional blenders or mixers, handheld immersion blenders offer unparalleled control and precision. Their compact size and ergonomic design allow artisans to maneuver through ingredients with ease, ensuring thorough blending without the need for multiple appliances or excessive cleanup.

Emulsification is the magic that transforms disparate ingredients into cohesive skincare treasures. With the flick of a switch, handheld immersion blenders effortlessly combine oil and water-based components, coaxing them into harmonious union. The result? Silky-smooth creams, luxurious lotions, and velvety serums that glide effortlessly onto the skin, delivering nourishment and hydration with every application.

One of the greatest strengths of handheld immersion blenders lies in their versatility. Whether whipping up a lightweight moisturizer or a rich, indulgent balm, these handy devices adapt to the unique needs of each formulation, ensuring consistent results every time. From emulsifying botanical oils to dispersing aqueous extracts, their prowess knows no bounds.

In addition to their blending capabilities, handheld immersion blenders excel in creating stable emulsions that resist separation over time. By thoroughly incorporating oil and water molecules, they prevent the dreaded "oil slick" or "watery puddle" that can plague poorly emulsified formulations, ensuring that skincare products maintain their integrity and efficacy.

Beyond functionality, handheld immersion blenders offer practical benefits that streamline the formulation process. Their compact size and cordless operation make them ideal for small-scale batch production, allowing artisans to experiment with new recipes without the constraints of bulky machinery or limited workspace.

Moreover, handheld immersion blenders are easy to clean and maintain, with detachable blending attachments that can be washed with soap and water or conveniently stored for future use. This simplicity not only saves time but also promotes hygiene, ensuring that each batch of skincare is crafted with the utmost care and cleanliness.

For DIY skincare enthusiasts, handheld immersion blenders represent more than just a tool; they are a symbol of creativity and innovation. With their help, artisans can transform humble ingredients into luxurious formulations that rival those found in high-end spas and boutiques, empowering individuals to take control of their skincare journey with confidence and flair.

The handheld immersion blender is a must-have tool for any serious DIY skincare crafter. Its ability to emulsify oil and water-based ingredients with precision and ease opens up a world of possibilities, allowing artisans to create bespoke formulations that cater to their unique skincare needs. With a handheld immersion blender in hand, the only limit to skincare creativity is imagination.

Crafting Comfort
The Role of Heat-Safe Containers

When it comes to DIY skincare formulation, every detail counts, especially when it involves heat-sensitive ingredients. Heat-safe containers, such as those made of glass or stainless steel, play a pivotal role in ensuring the safe and effective melting and heating of various skincare ingredients. From double boilers to heat-resistant beakers, these containers provide a reliable and controlled environment for crafting luxurious skincare concoctions.

At the heart of skincare formulation lies the delicate art of melting and heating ingredients to achieve the desired consistency and texture. Heat-safe containers act as the guardians of this process, offering a secure vessel for gently melting oils, waxes, and butters without compromising their integrity or efficacy.

Double boilers are a staple in the skincare artisan's toolkit, providing a foolproof method for indirect heating that minimizes the risk of scorching or overheating delicate ingredients. By placing a heat-safe container filled with ingredients atop a pot of simmering water, artisans can melt oils and waxes slowly and evenly, ensuring a smooth and uniform texture.

Heat-resistant beakers are another essential component of the DIY skincare workstation, offering a versatile and convenient option for heating and mixing ingredients. Made from durable materials like borosilicate glass or stainless steel, these containers can withstand high temperatures without warping or leaching harmful chemicals into formulations.

The beauty of heat-safe containers lies in their ability to provide a controlled environment for heating ingredients, allowing artisans to tailor the temperature to the specific requirements of each formulation. Whether melting shea butter for a nourishing body balm or heating water for a hydrating facial mist, these containers offer the precision and reliability needed for successful skincare crafting.

In addition to their functional benefits, heat-safe containers also offer practical advantages in terms of hygiene and cleanliness. Unlike plastic containers, which can degrade and leach chemicals when exposed to heat, glass and stainless steel containers are non-reactive and easy to sanitize, ensuring that skincare formulations remain pure and uncontaminated.

Furthermore, heat-safe containers are reusable and eco-friendly, reducing the need for single-use packaging and minimizing waste in the skincare formulation process. By investing in durable, long-lasting containers, artisans can minimize their environmental footprint while maximizing the longevity of their skincare crafting endeavors.

For DIY skincare enthusiasts, heat-safe containers are more than just vessels for ingredients; they are symbols of craftsmanship and care. With their help, artisans can transform raw materials into luxurious skincare formulations that rival commercial products in quality and efficacy, all from the comfort of their own homes.

4.2

Safety Measures
and Good Manufacturing Practices

Guarding Your Craft
The Importance of Protective Gear

In the world of DIY skincare formulation, safety should always take center stage. As artisans embark on their creative journeys, it's crucial to prioritize protective gear to safeguard against potential hazards. From gloves and aprons to safety goggles, these essential tools serve as the first line of defense when handling raw ingredients, particularly potent substances like concentrated essential oils or caustic compounds such as lye.

Gloves stand as the cornerstone of protective gear, providing a barrier between the skin and potentially harmful ingredients. When working with raw materials that can irritate or cause allergic reactions, such as essential oils or acidic solutions, gloves offer essential protection against direct contact, minimizing the risk of skin irritation, burns, or other adverse reactions.

Aprons serve as a shield against spills, splashes, and stains, keeping clothing clean and protected during the skincare crafting process. Whether it's mixing potent formulations or handling messy ingredients, aprons provide an additional layer of defense against accidental exposure, ensuring artisans can focus on their craft without worrying about damaging their attire.

Safety goggles play a critical role in safeguarding the eyes from splashes, vapors, or airborne particles that may pose a risk during skincare formulation. When working with volatile substances or handling ingredients that can release irritating fumes, such as certain acids or solvents, safety goggles offer essential eye protection, reducing the risk of injury or irritation.

It's important to select gloves, aprons, and safety goggles that are specifically designed for use in skincare formulation to ensure optimal protection and comfort. Disposable nitrile gloves are a popular choice due to their durability, flexibility, and resistance to chemicals, while reusable rubber or latex gloves offer a more sustainable option for artisans who prefer a washable option.

When choosing an apron, opt for materials that are water-resistant and easy to clean, such as vinyl or polyester, to provide maximum coverage and protection against spills and splatters. Look for aprons with adjustable straps and secure closures to ensure a comfortable and secure fit throughout the skincare crafting process.

Similarly, select safety goggles with shatterproof lenses and a snug, adjustable fit to provide maximum coverage and protection for the eyes. Anti-fog coatings can also help maintain visibility and clarity, especially when working in humid or steamy environments.

In addition to wearing protective gear, it's essential to practice good manufacturing practices (GMP) to minimize the risk of contamination and ensure the safety and efficacy of skincare formulations. This includes maintaining a clean and organized workspace, properly labeling and storing ingredients, and following standardized procedures for measuring, mixing, and handling raw materials.

Creating a Sanitary Haven
The Importance of a Clean Work Surface

The significance of a pristine work surface cannot be overstated. A clean and sanitized workspace serves as the foundation upon which safe and effective formulations are built, offering assurance of purity and quality throughout the skincare crafting process. By upholding meticulous standards of cleanliness and organization, artisans can mitigate the risk of contamination and uphold the integrity of their creations.

At the heart of a clean work surface lies the commitment to maintaining a sanitary environment, devoid of contaminants and clutter. This entails regularly disinfecting surfaces and equipment to eradicate bacteria, viruses, and other harmful microorganisms that may compromise the safety and efficacy of skincare formulations. By adopting stringent sanitation practices, artisans can instill confidence in the purity and reliability of their products.

Organization is key to fostering a clean and efficient workspace. By establishing designated areas for ingredient storage, mixing, and packaging, artisans can streamline their workflow and minimize the risk of cross-contamination. Proper labeling of ingredients and containers further enhances clarity and ensures accuracy in skincare formulation, reducing the likelihood of errors or mixups.

In addition to cleanliness and organization, ventilation plays a pivotal role in maintaining a healthy work environment. Adequate airflow helps dissipate airborne particles and fumes, reducing the concentration of potentially harmful substances in the workspace. Proper ventilation is particularly crucial when working with volatile ingredients or chemicals that may emit strong odors or vapors.

Regular maintenance of equipment and tools is essential for preserving their functionality and integrity. This includes cleaning and disinfecting mixing bowls, spatulas, and other utensils after each use to prevent the buildup of residue or contaminants. Sharpening blades and replacing worn-out components ensures optimal performance and reduces the risk of accidents or injuries during skincare formulation.

Adhering to good manufacturing practices (GMP) is fundamental to maintaining a clean work surface and upholding product safety and quality standards. This involves following standardized procedures for cleaning and sanitizing equipment, storing ingredients properly, and maintaining meticulous records of production processes. By embracing GMP principles, artisans can instill trust in their customers and uphold the reputation of their skincare brand.

A clean work surface serves as the cornerstone of safe and effective skincare formulation. By prioritizing cleanliness, organization, and ventilation, artisans can create an environment conducive to product purity and integrity. Through adherence to good manufacturing practices and regular maintenance of equipment, artisans can uphold the highest standards of quality and safety in their skincare creations, fostering confidence and trust among consumers.

Sanitizing Equipment and Containers
Essential Techniques

Maintaining proper sanitation practices is paramount when crafting homemade skincare products to guarantee product safety and efficacy. Sterilizing skincare equipment and containers is vital to prevent bacterial contamination and preserve product integrity. Fortunately, several techniques can be employed for effective sanitization, each with its unique advantages and considerations.

Hydrogen peroxide emerges as a readily available and easy-to-use disinfectant for sanitizing skincare equipment and containers. With its potent antimicrobial properties, hydrogen peroxide effectively kills bacteria, viruses, and fungi on surfaces. However, caution must be exercised, as it may not be suitable for certain materials like plastics, which can suffer damage or discoloration upon prolonged exposure. Additionally, hydrogen peroxide residue may persist if not thoroughly rinsed.

UV sterilization devices offer a convenient and efficient method for sanitizing skincare tools and containers. Harnessing UV light, particularly UV-C, these devices possess germicidal properties capable of destroying microorganisms. While UV sterilizers are user-friendly and require minimal effort, they may struggle to penetrate shadowed areas effectively, potentially leading to incomplete sterilization. Moreover, prolonged UV exposure can degrade certain materials over time, necessitating careful consideration of equipment compatibility.

Ozone generators present another compelling option, producing ozone gas—an effective oxidizing agent that eradicates bacteria, viruses, and fungi. This sterilization method is not only potent but also chemical-free, aligning with eco-conscious practices. However, the initial investment required for ozone generators can be significant, and proper ventilation is essential to mitigate exposure to high levels of ozone gas, which can pose respiratory risks.

Boiling remains a straightforward and cost-effective method for sterilizing skincare equipment and containers at home. By subjecting items to high temperatures, boiling effectively eliminates microorganisms. Although suitable for heat-resistant materials, boiling may not be ideal for plastics and rubber, as it can cause deformation or degradation. Furthermore, boiling necessitates ample water and may prove time-consuming, particularly for large batches of equipment.

Autoclaving stands out as a professional-grade sterilization technique that ensures thorough microorganism eradication. This process involves subjecting skincare tools and containers to high-pressure steam at temperatures exceeding the boiling point. While highly effective, autoclaving demands specialized equipment and may not be feasible for home use due to its cost and complexity.

Industrial sanitization products such as **isopropyl alcohol** and **chlorine bleach** are renowned for their effectiveness in sterilizing skincare equipment and containers. These potent agents boast broad-spectrum antimicrobial activity, readily available and accessible. However, they can be harsh on certain materials and necessitate proper ventilation and protective gear during use. Additionally, chlorine bleach may leave behind residue and has the potential to discolor fabrics and surfaces.

Maintaining proper sanitation practices is imperative for the safety and efficacy of homemade skincare products. By embracing effective sanitization techniques such as hydrogen peroxide, UV sterilization, ozone sterilization, boiling, autoclaving, and industrial sanitization products, individuals can minimize the risk of bacterial contamination and craft high-quality skincare formulations with confidence. Each method offers unique benefits and considerations, providing flexibility in selecting the most suitable option based on specific needs and preferences.

Keeping Track and Labeling
A Must-Have for DIY Skincare Crafters

When it comes to crafting your own skincare goodies, two essential practices often get overlooked but are absolutely critical: keeping detailed batch records and labeling your products accurately. These steps are not just about ticking boxes; they're about transparency, accountability, and most importantly, your safety and that of your customers. Let's dive into why batch records and labeling matter so much and how they can make a real difference in your skincare game.

First up, batch records are like your skincare formula's diary. They document everything from the ingredients you use to when and how you made the product. It's not just a record-keeping chore; it's your secret weapon for consistency and quality control. With detailed batch records, you can track what works (and what doesn't), replicate successful formulas, and catch any issues before they become big problems.

But batch records aren't just about your peace of mind; they're also crucial for playing by the rules. If you ever get audited or inspected, having solid batch records shows that you're following the Good Manufacturing Practices (GMP) and other regulations. It's your golden ticket to proving that your products are safe, reliable, and made with care.

Now, let's talk about labeling – your product's first impression. Labeling isn't just about slapping on a name; it's about giving your customers the lowdown on what they're putting on their skin. Your labels should be like a mini user manual, with clear ingredient lists, directions for use, and any warnings for sensitive souls. It's not just about being transparent; it's about empowering your customers to make informed choices.

Accurate labeling isn't just about playing nice; it's about building trust. When your customers see that you've laid it all out on the label – no hidden nasties or confusing jargon – they'll know they can count on you. It's about more than just selling a product; it's about building a relationship built on honesty and integrity.

And let's not forget about traceability. If something goes wrong (heaven forbid!), having those batch records on hand can be a lifesaver. Whether it's a quality issue or a safety concern, being able to trace back to the source quickly and efficiently can mean the difference between a hiccup and a disaster.

So, whether you're whipping up skincare treats for yourself or selling them to others, don't skimp on the record-keeping and labeling. It's not just about following the rules; it's about showing that you care – about your craft, about your customers, and about doing things right. With meticulous batch records and clear labeling, you're not just making skincare; you're making a statement – one of transparency, accountability, and trust.

4.3

Tips for Storing and Preserving Homemade Products

Preserving Potency
The Power of Air-Tight Containers

How you store your precious creations can make all the difference in their effectiveness and longevity. That's where air-tight containers swoop in as unsung heroes. These opaque, tightly sealed vessels, typically crafted from glass or PET plastic, act as guardians, shielding your homemade skincare concoctions from their sworn enemies: light, air, and moisture. Let's unpack why air-tight containers are the go-to choice for savvy skincare crafters and how they can help preserve the potency of your prized formulations.

First off, let's talk about protection from the elements. Light, air, and moisture are the trifecta of skincare spoilage, causing ingredients to degrade, lose potency, and even turn rancid. Air-tight containers create a fortress against these threats, keeping your precious potions safe and sound until they're ready to work their magic on your skin.

But it's not just about warding off environmental foes; it's also about maximizing shelf life and stability. Exposure to light and air can accelerate oxidation, causing ingredients like oils and botanical extracts to go bad faster. By sealing them away in air-tight containers, you're giving them the best chance at staying fresh and potent for longer, so you can enjoy the full benefits of your creations down to the last drop.

Now, let's talk about the materials themselves. Glass and PET plastic are the MVPs of air-tight containers for several reasons. Glass is non-reactive, meaning it won't interact with your skincare ingredients or leach harmful chemicals into your formulations. Plus, it's recyclable and infinitely reusable, making it an eco-friendly choice for conscious crafters. PET plastic, on the other hand, is lightweight, shatter-resistant, and more affordable, making it a practical option for those on a budget or concerned about breakage.

Another key advantage of air-tight containers is their versatility. Whether you're storing creams, serums, oils, or masks, there's an air-tight container to suit every need. From jars and bottles to pumps and sprayers, these containers come in a variety of shapes, sizes, and designs to accommodate all your skincare creations – big or small, thick or thin.

But perhaps the most underrated benefit of air-tight containers is their convenience. With their snug-fitting lids and leak-proof seals, they're the perfect travel companions, ensuring your skincare essentials stay safe and spill-free wherever you go. No more worrying about messy leaks or broken bottles – just grab and go with confidence, knowing your skincare stash is securely tucked away.

Air-tight containers are the unsung heroes of DIY skincare, offering a simple yet effective solution for preserving the potency and stability of your homemade creations. With their ability to shield against light, air, and moisture, these containers ensure your skincare goodies stay fresh, potent, and ready to work their magic whenever you need them. So, whether you're a seasoned skincare crafter or just dipping your toes into the world of DIY beauty, don't underestimate the power of air-tight containers – they're a game-changer for preserving the integrity of your skincare treasures.

Keeping it Cool
The Importance of Proper Storage Conditions

What happens after you've crafted your perfect potion is just as crucial as the formulation process itself. Enter storage conditions – the unsung heroes of skincare longevity. Properly storing your finished products in the right environment can mean the difference between a potent elixir and a lackluster potion. Let's delve into why storing skincare creations in a cool, dry place away from direct sunlight and extreme temperatures is essential for maintaining their efficacy and freshness.

First and foremost, let's talk about temperature. Skincare ingredients, particularly natural ones, can be sensitive souls. Exposure to extreme temperatures – whether scorching heat or freezing cold – can wreak havoc on their stability and effectiveness. Storing products in a cool, stable environment helps prevent ingredients from degrading, separating, or losing potency, ensuring they deliver the results you're after.

But it's not just about temperature; humidity plays a role too. Moisture is the arch-nemesis of skincare formulations, capable of causing mold, bacterial growth, and product spoilage. By keeping products in a dry environment, you're safeguarding them against these potential pitfalls, prolonging their shelf life and ensuring they remain safe and hygienic for use.

Next up, let's talk about sunlight. While sunshine might be nature's way of bringing warmth and light, it's not always a friend to skincare products. UV radiation can degrade certain ingredients, particularly those sensitive to light, like vitamin C and retinol, leading to reduced effectiveness and potential skin irritation. Storing products away from direct sunlight – whether in opaque containers or tucked away in a drawer – helps protect them from UV damage, preserving their potency and integrity.

But it's not just about avoiding the bad stuff; it's also about maximizing the good. Proper storage conditions can enhance the efficacy and longevity of your skincare creations, ensuring you get the most bang for your buck. By investing a little extra care in how you store your products, you can extend their shelf life, maintain their freshness, and reap the full benefits of their potent ingredients.

So, where's the best place to store your skincare treasures? A cool, dark place is your best bet – think a cabinet or drawer away from heat sources like radiators or ovens. Avoid storing products in the bathroom, where fluctuating temperatures and high humidity levels can spell trouble for their stability. Instead, opt for a dedicated skincare storage area in a cool, dry room, where your products can thrive.

Proper storage conditions are the unsung heroes of skincare longevity, ensuring your precious potions remain potent and effective for longer. By storing products in a cool, dry place away from direct sunlight and extreme temperatures, you're safeguarding their efficacy and freshness, ensuring they deliver the results you desire. So, whether you're a skincare enthusiast or a DIY aficionado, don't overlook the importance of proper storage – your skin will thank you for it.

Keeping Skincare Fresh
A Guide to Preserving Homemade Potions

Preservation in DIY skincare mirrors the delicate balance of maintaining a thriving ecosystem in the classroom, where each component plays a crucial role in sustaining the overall integrity and efficacy of the formulation. Let's embark on an enlightening journey to uncover the intricate mechanisms of preservation and delve into practical strategies for safeguarding homemade skincare creations.

Understanding the Ingredients is akin to tailoring teaching methods to suit diverse learning styles. Skincare enthusiasts must grasp the properties of each ingredient to effectively preserve their formulations. For instance, water-based products are more prone to microbial growth, necessitating stronger preservation methods compared to oil-based ones. By comprehending ingredient nuances, creators can devise targeted preservation strategies tailored to their formulations.

The debate between Natural vs. Synthetic Preservatives mirrors the dichotomy between traditional and progressive teaching methods. Skincare enthusiasts often grapple with choosing between synthetic preservatives like parabens and phenoxyethanol, which offer potent antimicrobial properties, and natural alternatives such as grapefruit seed extract and rosemary extract, which align with eco-conscious values. Finding a balance between the two allows for comprehensive protection without compromising product safety.

Finding Balance, much like educators striking a balance between fostering creativity and maintaining discipline, is essential in preservation methods. Combining synthetic and natural preservatives ensures robust protection while minimizing the use of synthetic chemicals. For example, blending benzyl alcohol with plant-derived antioxidants offers effective preservation while retaining product integrity.

Storage Best Practices extend beyond formulation to encompass storage conditions. Similar to safeguarding educational materials, storing skincare products in cool, dark places shields them from environmental factors that could compromise integrity. Airtight containers made of opaque materials like amber glass or PET plastic provide an additional layer of protection against air and light exposure.

Educating Consumers is vital for fostering trust and confidence, akin to transparent communication in the classroom. Clear labeling empowers consumers to make informed decisions about skincare products. By educating consumers about proper storage and usage, creators cultivate a community of informed skincare enthusiasts.

Practical Examples illustrate preservation challenges and solutions:

- Formulating a water-based facial serum requires robust preservation to prevent microbial contamination. Incorporating broad-spectrum preservatives like phenoxyethanol and ethylhexylglycerin ensures product safety while preserving its natural appeal.

- Crafting an oil-based body balm presents different preservation challenges. Adding natural antioxidants such as vitamin E oil and rosemary extract extends the formulation's shelf life and protects it from oxidative rancidity.

- Educating consumers about proper storage empowers them to prolong their DIY skincare products' efficacy. Practical tips foster accountability and responsibility among consumers.

Preservation in DIY skincare requires a multifaceted approach. Understanding ingredient nuances, finding balance between natural and synthetic preservatives, practicing proper storage, and educating consumers are essential. By adopting practical strategies, skincare enthusiasts can ensure the longevity and effectiveness of their creations while fostering transparency and empowerment within the skincare community.

Safeguarding Skincare
The Importance of Product Testing

Product testing serves as a vital checkpoint in the journey of DIY skincare formulation, providing assurance of the safety, efficacy, and quality of homemade products. Similar to quality assurance protocols in industrial manufacturing, product testing involves a series of rigorous assessments aimed at evaluating the stability, microbial purity, and overall performance of skincare formulations.

Stability testing is akin to subjecting skincare products to a battery of stress tests, simulating real-world conditions to assess their resilience and shelf life. For instance, a homemade moisturizer may undergo stability testing to evaluate its performance when exposed to fluctuating temperatures, light exposure, and air. This process helps creators identify potential issues such as ingredient separation, color changes, or texture variations, ensuring that the product remains stable and effective over time.

Microbial testing, on the other hand, focuses on verifying the absence of harmful microorganisms in skincare formulations. Water-based products, in particular, are susceptible to microbial contamination, which can compromise product safety and pose health risks to consumers. Microbial testing involves culturing the product to detect the presence of bacteria, yeast, and mold, ensuring that it meets stringent microbial purity standards.

By conducting comprehensive stability and microbial testing, creators can validate the safety and quality of their DIY skincare formulations. This not only ensures compliance with regulatory standards but also instills confidence in consumers regarding the efficacy and safety of the products they use on their skin. Ultimately, product testing is essential for maintaining transparency, integrity, and trust within the DIY skincare community.

For example, consider a homemade facial serum formulated with potent botanical extracts and antioxidants. Before bringing it to market or sharing it with others, the creator may subject the serum to stability testing to assess its resilience to environmental stressors such as temperature fluctuations and light exposure. Additionally, microbial testing may be conducted to confirm the absence of harmful pathogens, ensuring that the serum remains safe for daily use.

Moreover, product testing serves as a valuable tool for continuous improvement and refinement of DIY skincare formulations. By analyzing the results of stability and microbial testing, creators can identify areas for optimization and fine-tuning, leading to the development of more effective and reliable skincare products. This iterative process not only enhances the safety and efficacy of formulations but also demonstrates a commitment to ongoing quality assurance and consumer satisfaction.

In conclusion, product testing plays a multifaceted role in DIY skincare formulation, encompassing stability assessment, microbial verification, and quality control measures. By subjecting formulations to rigorous testing protocols, creators can ensure the safety, efficacy, and integrity of their homemade skincare products, thereby fostering trust and confidence within the skincare community.

Chapter 5

Basic DIY Skincare Recipes for Beginners

Now that you've unlocked the secrets of your skin type and assembled your alchemist's toolkit, it's time to embark on the most exciting phase of this journey – crafting your very own DIY skincare recipes! This chapter unveils a collection of simple yet effective formulations, perfect for those embarking on their natural skincare adventure. Designed with readily available ingredients and beginner-friendly techniques, these recipes empower you to create personalized solutions that cater to your unique needs.

But before we dive into the bubbling concoctions, remember, formulating your own skincare is an art and a science! Don't be afraid to experiment and adjust these recipes to your liking. Here are some helpful tips to guide you on your DIY journey:

- *Start Slow*: Begin with a single recipe and patch-test it on a small area of your inner arm before applying it to your entire face. This helps identify any potential sensitivities.

- *Listen to Your Skin*: Pay close attention to how your skin reacts to each ingredient. If you experience any irritation, discontinue use and adjust the recipe accordingly.

- *Embrace the Fresh Factor*: Since most DIY products lack preservatives, it's best to make them in small batches and use them within a week or two.

- *Hygiene is Key*: Always sterilize your jars and utensils before whipping up your concoctions to prevent bacterial growth.

Most Importantly, Have Fun! Experimentation is half the charm of DIY skincare. Don't be afraid to get creative and personalize these recipes to reflect your unique preferences and the ever-changing needs of your skin.

With these guidelines in mind, get ready to unleash your inner alchemist and embark on a journey of creating personalized skincare magic!

A Recap of Common DIY Skincare Ingredients

In next chapters, we will delve into the world of DIY natural skincare ingredients, exploring the diverse range of options available to create personalized skincare formulations. From carrier oils to essential oils and everything in between, discover the power of nature's bounty for your skincare routine.

Carrier Oils: Jojoba oil, coconut oil, almond oil, and olive oil serve as the foundation for many DIY skincare recipes. These oils provide moisturizing properties and serve as base oils for diluting essential oils.

Essential Oils: Essential oils are concentrated extracts derived from plants and offer various therapeutic benefits. Lavender, tea tree, rosemary, and chamomile essential oils are popular choices for their anti-inflammatory, antimicrobial, and soothing properties.

Shea Butter: Shea butter is a rich and nourishing butter extracted from the nuts of the shea tree. It is prized for its moisturizing and emollient qualities, making it an excellent choice for dry and damaged skin.

Cocoa Butter: Cocoa butter, derived from cocoa beans, is known for its hydrating properties and luxurious texture. It is commonly used in lip balms, body butters, and creams to soften and smooth the skin.

Beeswax: Beeswax is a natural thickening agent and emulsifier commonly used in balms, salves, and lotions. It creates a protective barrier on the skin while locking in moisture, making it particularly beneficial for dry and sensitive skin.

Aloe Vera Gel: Aloe vera gel is renowned for its soothing and hydrating properties, making it a popular ingredient in skincare products. It helps to calm irritation, reduce inflammation, and promote healing, making it suitable for all skin types.

Hyaluronic Acid Serum: Hyaluronic acid serum is a hydrating skincare product that helps to plump and moisturize the skin. It is commonly used to reduce the appearance of fine lines and wrinkles and improve skin texture and tone.

Clay: Various clays, such as bentonite, kaolin, and French green clay, are used in skincare products for their detoxifying and purifying effects. They help to draw out impurities, unclog pores, and absorb excess oil, making them ideal for oily and acne-prone skin.

Honey: Honey is a natural humectant with antibacterial properties, making it an excellent ingredient for moisturizing and clarifying the skin. It helps to retain moisture and promote a healthy complexion.

Oatmeal: Ground oats are prized for their gentle exfoliating properties and soothing effect on irritated or sensitive skin. They help to remove dead skin cells, calm inflammation, and promote healing.

Rosewater: Rosewater is a refreshing toner distilled from rose petals. It helps to balance the skin's pH, hydrate, and soothe inflammation, making it suitable for all skin types.

Where to Find These Ingredients

Health Food Stores: Look for natural and organic skincare ingredients at health food stores like Whole Foods Market or local co-ops.

Online Retailers: Websites such as Amazon, Mountain Rose Herbs, and Etsy offer a wide range of natural skincare ingredients.

Farmers Markets: Some farmers markets may have vendors selling locally sourced and organic ingredients like honey, beeswax, and herbal extracts.

Specialty Stores: Specialty stores focused on natural living and wellness often carry a selection of skincare ingredients.

Gardens and Farms: Grow your own herbs, flowers, and botanicals for use in DIY skincare or purchase them directly from local farmers.

Hyaluronic Acid Serum: Where to Find It

Beauty Stores: Sephora, Ulta Beauty, and other specialty beauty retailers carry hyaluronic acid serums from various brands.

Drugstores: Brands like CeraVe, Neutrogena, and The Ordinary offer affordable options that can be found at drugstore chains like CVS and Walgreens.

Online Retailers: Amazon, eBay, and individual brand websites offer a wide selection of hyaluronic acid serums tailored to different skin types and concerns.

When purchasing ingredients, prioritize quality and authenticity. Look for organic, sustainably sourced options whenever possible to ensure the highest quality skincare products. With these natural ingredients, you can create personalized skincare formulations tailored to your specific needs and preferences, all while harnessing the power of nature

5.1

Gentle Cleansers and Makeup Removers

Soothing Milk Cleanser
A Nourishing DIY Recipe for Gentle Skincare

Indulge in the soothing embrace of nature with our homemade Soothing Milk Cleanser. Crafted from wholesome ingredients like almond milk, honey, and oatmeal, this gentle cleanser offers a nourishing cleanse that leaves your skin feeling refreshed and rejuvenated.

Ingredients

- 1/2 cup almond milk

- 2 tablespoons honey

- 2 tablespoons finely ground oatmeal

Preparation Instructions

- In a clean mixing bowl, combine the almond milk and honey. Stir until the honey is thoroughly mixed with the almond milk.

- Gradually add the finely ground oatmeal to the mixture, stirring continuously to create a smooth paste.

- Transfer the mixture to a clean, airtight container for storage.

Usage Instructions

- Dampen your face with lukewarm water.

- Apply a small amount of the Soothing Milk Cleanser to your fingertips.

- Gently massage the cleanser onto your skin using circular motions.

- Allow the cleanser to sit on your skin for a few moments.

- Rinse thoroughly with lukewarm water and pat your skin dry with a soft towel.

- Follow up with your favorite toner and moisturizer.

Benefits for Different Skin Types

- Dry or Sensitive Skin: The Soothing Milk Cleanser offers a gentle cleanse while hydrating and soothing dry or sensitive skin.

- Oily or Acne-Prone Skin: Despite its creamy texture, this cleanser is non-comedogenic and helps remove excess oil and impurities without clogging pores.

Storage and Shelf Life

Store the Soothing Milk Cleanser in a clean, airtight container in a cool, dry place away from direct sunlight. It can typically be kept for up to one to two weeks. However, it's best to make smaller batches and use them within a shorter timeframe for freshness and effectiveness.

Gentle Micellar Water Recipe
A Refreshing DIY Makeup Remover

Discover the gentle yet effective power of our homemade Micellar Water. Formulated with micellar water, witch hazel, and aloe vera gel, this refreshing cleanser effortlessly removes makeup and impurities while soothing sensitive skin.

Ingredients

- 1/2 cup micellar water

- 1/4 cup witch hazel

- 2 tablespoons aloe vera gel

Preparation Instructions

- In a clean mixing bowl, combine the micellar water and witch hazel.

- Add the aloe vera gel to the mixture and stir well until thoroughly combined.

- Transfer the micellar water solution to a clean, airtight container for storage.

Usage Instructions

- Shake the bottle of Micellar Water to ensure all ingredients are well mixed.

- Apply a small amount of Micellar Water to a cotton pad or reusable cloth.

- Gently swipe the soaked cotton pad over your face, eyes, and lips to remove makeup and impurities.

- Repeat as needed until your skin feels clean and refreshed.

- There is no need to rinse off the Micellar Water, but you can follow up with your favorite moisturizer if desired.

Benefits for Different Skin Types

- Sensitive Skin: The gentle formula of Micellar Water, combined with soothing aloe vera gel, makes it perfect for sensitive skin types prone to irritation.

- Quick Makeup Removal: Micellar Water effectively lifts away makeup, dirt, and oil without the need for harsh rubbing, making it ideal for quick and convenient makeup removal.

Storage and Shelf Life:

Store the Micellar Water in a clean, airtight container in a cool, dry place away from direct sunlight. It can typically be kept for up to one to two weeks. However, for optimal freshness and effectiveness, it's best to make smaller batches and use them within a shorter timeframe.

5.2

Hydrating Toners
and Refreshing Mists

Hydrating Rosewater Toner Recipe
Nourish and Balance Your Skin

Indulge in the luxurious essence of roses with our homemade Rosewater Toner. This refreshing toner, enriched with rosewater, witch hazel, and glycerin, hydrates, soothes, and balances the skin's pH after cleansing, leaving your complexion refreshed and revitalized.

Ingredients

- 1/2 cup rosewater

- 1/4 cup witch hazel

- 1 tablespoon glycerin

Preparation Instructions:

- In a clean mixing bowl, combine the rosewater and witch hazel.

- Add the glycerin to the mixture and stir well until thoroughly combined.

- Transfer the rosewater toner solution to a clean, airtight container for storage.

Usage Instructions

- After cleansing your face, apply a small amount of Rosewater Toner to a cotton pad or reusable cloth.

- Gently swipe the soaked cotton pad over your face and neck, avoiding the eye area.

- Allow the toner to dry naturally on your skin.

• Follow up with your favorite moisturizer or serum for added hydration.

Benefits for Different Skin Types

• Hydration: Rosewater and glycerin help hydrate the skin, making this toner suitable for dry and dehydrated skin types.

• Soothing: Witch hazel has soothing properties that can help calm inflammation and redness, making this toner ideal for sensitive or irritated skin.

• pH Balancing: The combination of ingredients in this toner helps balance the skin's pH levels, promoting a healthy complexion for all skin types.

Storage and Shelf Life

Store the Rosewater Toner in a clean, airtight container in a cool, dry place away from direct sunlight. It can typically be kept for up to one to two weeks. However, for optimal freshness and effectiveness, it's best to make smaller batches and use them within a shorter timeframe.

Cooling Cucumber Mint Facial Mist Recipe
Refresh and Revitalize Your Skin

Experience a burst of freshness with our homemade Cucumber Mint Facial Mist. This cooling and invigorating mist, infused with cucumber juice, mint leaves, and green tea extract, instantly refreshes and revitalizes tired skin, leaving you feeling rejuvenated and radiant.

Ingredients

- 1/2 cup cucumber juice

- Handful of fresh mint leaves

- 1 teaspoon green tea extract

Preparation Instructions

- Begin by juicing half a cucumber to obtain approximately 1/2 cup of cucumber juice.

- In a blender or food processor, combine the cucumber juice and fresh mint leaves.

- Blend the mixture until the mint leaves are finely chopped and incorporated into the cucumber juice.

- Strain the mixture through a fine-mesh sieve or cheesecloth to remove any solid particles.

- Add the green tea extract to the strained cucumber and mint mixture and stir well to combine.

- Transfer the facial mist solution to a clean, empty spray bottle for storage.

Usage Instructions:

• Shake the Cucumber Mint Facial Mist bottle well before each use to ensure the ingredients are evenly distributed.

• Close your eyes and hold the bottle approximately 6-8 inches away from your face.

• Spritz the mist lightly and evenly over your face and neck, avoiding the eye area.

• Allow the mist to air dry or gently pat it into your skin with clean fingertips.

• Use the facial mist as needed throughout the day to refresh and hydrate your skin, especially during hot weather or after physical activity.

Benefits for Different Skin Types:

• Refreshing: Cucumber juice provides a cooling sensation, making this facial mist perfect for refreshing and revitalizing tired or overheated skin.

• Invigorating: Mint leaves impart a refreshing and invigorating aroma while also providing a soothing sensation to the skin, making this mist suitable for all skin types, including sensitive skin.

• Antioxidant-Rich: Green tea extract is rich in antioxidants, which help protect the skin from environmental stressors and promote a healthy complexion.

Storage and Shelf Life

Store the Cucumber Mint Facial Mist in the refrigerator to prolong its freshness and enhance its cooling effect. It can typically be kept for up to one to two weeks. However, for optimal freshness and effectiveness, it's best to make smaller batches and use them within a shorter timeframe.

5.3

Moisturizers
for Day and Night

Luxurious Nourishing Face Cream
Hydrate and Soften Your Skin

Indulge your skin with our sumptuous Nourishing Face Cream, a rich and moisturizing blend of shea butter, jojoba oil, and vitamin E oil. Designed to hydrate and soften dry skin, this decadent cream is perfect for nighttime use, providing intense nourishment while you sleep.

Ingredients

- 1/4 cup shea butter

- 2 tablespoons jojoba oil

- 1 teaspoon vitamin E oil

Preparation Instructions

- In a double boiler or heat-safe bowl set over a pot of simmering water, melt the shea butter until it becomes a liquid.

- Once the shea butter is melted, remove it from the heat and stir in the jojoba oil and vitamin E oil until well combined.

- Allow the mixture to cool slightly, but not solidify completely.

- Transfer the mixture to a clean, airtight container or jar for storage.

Usage Instructions

- After cleansing and toning your face, scoop a small amount of the Nourishing Face Cream onto your fingertips.

- Gently massage the cream into your skin using upward circular motions, focusing on areas prone to dryness.

- Allow the cream to absorb fully before applying any additional skincare products or makeup.

- For best results, use the Nourishing Face Cream as part of your nighttime skincare routine to provide deep hydration and replenishment while you sleep.

Benefits for Different Skin Types

- Hydrating: Shea butter and jojoba oil are deeply moisturizing ingredients that help hydrate and soften dry skin, making this cream ideal for those with dry or dehydrated skin.

- Nourishing: Vitamin E oil is rich in antioxidants and helps nourish and protect the skin from environmental damage, promoting a healthy and radiant complexion.

- Gentle: The gentle formulation of this face cream makes it suitable for most skin types, including sensitive skin, providing luxurious hydration without irritation.

Storage and Shelf Life

Store the Nourishing Face Cream in a cool, dry place away from direct sunlight to maintain its freshness and efficacy. It can typically be kept for up to three to six months. However, for optimal results, it's best to use the cream within a few months of preparation.

Lightweight Gel Moisturizer
Soothing and refreshing skin

Experience lightweight hydration with our Gel Moisturizer, a non-greasy blend of aloe vera gel, hyaluronic acid, and cucumber extract. Designed to hydrate and soothe oily or combination skin, this refreshing gel is perfect for daytime use under makeup.

Ingredients:

- 1/4 cup aloe vera gel

- 1 tablespoon hyaluronic acid

- 1 teaspoon cucumber extract

Preparation Instructions

- Mix together 1/4 cup of aloe vera gel and 1 tablespoon of hyaluronic acid in a clean container.

- Add 1 teaspoon of cucumber extract and stir until well combined.

- Transfer the mixture to an airtight container or pump bottle for easy application.

Usage Instructions

- After cleansing and toning your face, apply a small amount of the Lightweight Gel Moisturizer onto your fingertips.

- Gently massage the gel into your skin using upward motions until fully absorbed.

- Allow the moisturizer to dry before applying sunscreen or makeup.

Benefits for Different Skin Types

- Hydrating: Aloe vera gel and hyaluronic acid provide lightweight hydration without feeling heavy or greasy, making it suitable for oily or combination skin.

- Soothing: Cucumber extract soothes and calms the skin, reducing redness and irritation.

- Non-Greasy: The lightweight gel texture absorbs quickly into the skin, leaving it feeling refreshed and hydrated without any residue.

Storage and Shelf Life

Store the Lightweight Gel Moisturizer in a cool, dry place away from direct sunlight. It can typically be kept for up to three to six months. For best results, use within a few months of preparation.

Chapter 6

Leveling Up:
Intermediate Skincare Formulations

Embark on an odyssey through the realms of advanced DIY skincare as we delve into intermediate-level formulations meticulously crafted to elevate your routine. In this chapter, we journey beyond the basics, exploring a diverse array of recipes tailored to address specific skin concerns and unlock transformative results.

Prepare to confront acne and blemishes head-on with our arsenal of targeted treatments. The Tea Tree Spot Treatment emerges as a potent elixir, blending tea tree essential oil, witch hazel, and aloe vera gel to combat inflammation, battle bacteria, and expedite the healing process.

Experience the purifying prowess of our Clay Mask for Congested Skin, a detoxifying blend of bentonite clay, activated charcoal, and tea tree oil engineered to draw out impurities, cleanse pores, and regulate oil production.

Seek rejuvenation with our selection of face masks and exfoliants. The Brightening Turmeric Mask offers a radiant boost, featuring turmeric, yogurt, and honey to illuminate dull skin and diminish dark spots. Meanwhile, our DIY Sugar Scrub, crafted from brown sugar, coconut oil, and citrus essential oils, promises to unveil a smoother, more luminous complexion.

Discover the science of skincare with our specialty serums, designed to brighten and firm. The Vitamin C Brightening Serum boasts a potent blend of vitamin C, hyaluronic acid, and botanical extracts to even skin tone, fade hyperpigmentation, and stimulate collagen production. And for deep hydration, the Hyaluronic Acid Hydrating Serum, infused with hyaluronic acid, panthenol, and cucumber extract, replenishes moisture, smooths fine lines, and restores elasticity.

Each formulation is accompanied by detailed instructions and tips for customization, ensuring tailored solutions for every skin type and preference. Embrace the journey as we unlock the potential of DIY skincare, transforming your routine into a realm of endless possibilities.

6.1

Targeted Treatments for Acne and Blemishes

Targeted Acne Relief
Tea Tree Spot Treatment

Combat pesky acne blemishes with our Tea Tree Spot Treatment, a powerful blend of tea tree essential oil, witch hazel, and aloe vera gel. This potent spot treatment is specifically formulated to reduce inflammation, fight bacteria, and promote the healing of acne blemishes, giving you clearer and healthier-looking skin.

Ingredients

- 1 tablespoon witch hazel

- 5 drops tea tree essential oil

- 1 tablespoon aloe vera gel

Preparation Instructions

- In a small bowl, combine the witch hazel and tea tree essential oil.

- Stir the mixture well to ensure the essential oil is evenly distributed.

- Add the aloe vera gel to the mixture and continue stirring until all ingredients are thoroughly combined.

- Transfer the spot treatment to a clean, airtight container for storage.

Usage Instructions

- Cleanse and dry the affected area of your skin before applying the spot treatment.

- Using a cotton swab or clean fingertip, apply a small amount of the Tea Tree Spot Treatment directly onto the blemish.

- Allow the spot treatment to dry completely before applying any additional skincare products or makeup.

- For best results, use the spot treatment twice daily, morning and night, until the blemish has healed.

Benefits for Different Skin Types

- Anti-inflammatory: Tea tree essential oil possesses anti-inflammatory properties that help reduce redness and inflammation associated with acne blemishes, making it suitable for all skin types, including sensitive skin.

- Antibacterial: The antimicrobial properties of tea tree oil and witch hazel work together to fight acne-causing bacteria, helping to prevent further breakouts and promote clearer skin.

- Soothing: Aloe vera gel helps soothe and calm irritated skin, providing relief from the discomfort often associated with acne blemishes, making this spot treatment gentle yet effective for all skin types.

Storage and Shelf Life

Store the Tea Tree Spot Treatment in a cool, dry place away from direct sunlight to maintain its potency and efficacy. It can typically be kept for up to three to six months. However, for optimal results, it's best to use the spot treatment within a few months of preparation.

Purify and Rejuvenate
Clay Mask for Congested Skin

Revitalize your skin with our Clay Mask for Congested Skin, a potent blend of bentonite clay, activated charcoal, and tea tree oil. This detoxifying mask is specially formulated to draw out impurities, unclog pores, and reduce excess oil production, leaving your skin feeling refreshed and rejuvenated.

Ingredients

- 1 tablespoon bentonite clay

- 1 teaspoon activated charcoal

- 3-4 drops tea tree essential oil

- Water or apple cider vinegar (ACV) for mixing

Preparation Instructions

- In a small bowl, combine the bentonite clay and activated charcoal.

- Add 3-4 drops of tea tree essential oil to the dry ingredients.

- Gradually add water or apple cider vinegar (ACV) to the mixture, stirring until a smooth paste is formed. Adjust the amount of liquid as needed to achieve the desired consistency.

- Once the mask reaches the desired consistency, it is ready to use.

Usage Instructions

- Start by cleansing your face to remove any dirt, oil, or makeup.

- Apply a thin, even layer of the Clay Mask for Congested Skin to your face, avoiding the delicate eye area and lips.

- Allow the mask to dry completely, typically for 10-15 minutes.

- Once dry, rinse off the mask thoroughly with warm water.

- Follow up with your favorite moisturizer to replenish hydration and lock in moisture.

Benefits for Different Skin Types

- Deep Cleansing: Bentonite clay and activated charcoal work synergistically to draw out impurities and toxins from the skin, making this mask ideal for congested and acne-prone skin types.

- Oil Balancing: The absorbent properties of bentonite clay help regulate excess oil production, while tea tree oil provides antibacterial benefits, making this mask suitable for oily and combination skin.

- Soothing: Despite its deep-cleansing properties, this mask is formulated with tea tree oil, which possesses soothing and anti-inflammatory properties, ensuring it remains gentle enough for sensitive skin types.

Storage and Shelf Life

Store any leftover Clay Mask for Congested Skin in a sealed container in a cool, dry place away from direct sunlight. When stored properly, the mask can typically be kept for up to one month. Be sure to mix the mask thoroughly before each use to ensure optimal efficacy

6.2

Rejuvenating Face Masks and Exfoliants

Illuminate Your Skin
Brightening Turmeric Mask

Unveil a radiant complexion with our Brightening Turmeric Mask, a rejuvenating blend of turmeric, yogurt, and honey. This revitalizing face mask is designed to brighten dull skin, fade dark spots, and promote a luminous glow, leaving your skin looking refreshed and revitalized.

Ingredients

- tablespoon turmeric powder
- 1 tablespoon plain yogurt
- 1 teaspoon honey

Preparation Instructions

- In a small bowl, combine the turmeric powder, plain yogurt, and honey.
- Stir the ingredients together until they form a smooth, uniform paste.

Usage Instructions:

- Begin by cleansing your face to remove any dirt, oil, or makeup.
- Apply a generous layer of the Brightening Turmeric Mask to your face, avoiding the delicate eye area and lips.
- Allow the mask to sit for 10-15 minutes to allow the ingredients to work their magic.

- After the designated time, gently rinse off the mask with lukewarm water, using gentle circular motions to exfoliate the skin as you remove the mask.

- Pat your skin dry with a soft towel and follow up with your favorite moisturizer to lock in hydration.

Benefits for Different Skin Types:

- Brightening: Turmeric is renowned for its brightening properties, making this mask ideal for dull, lackluster skin in need of a boost.

- Dark Spot Reduction: The combination of turmeric, yogurt, and honey works synergistically to fade dark spots and hyperpigmentation, promoting a more even-toned complexion.

- Hydration: Yogurt and honey are both hydrating ingredients that help replenish moisture and soothe the skin, making this mask suitable for dry and sensitive skin types.

Storage and Shelf Life:

Store any leftover Brightening Turmeric Mask in an airtight container in the refrigerator for up to one week. Due to the natural ingredients used in this mask, it is best to prepare fresh batches as needed to ensure optimal efficacy.

Revitalize Your Skin
DIY Sugar Scrub

Indulge in the ultimate pampering experience with our DIY Sugar Scrub, a luxurious blend of brown sugar, coconut oil, and citrus essential oils. This invigorating sugar scrub is designed to gently exfoliate the skin, sloughing away dead skin cells to reveal a smoother, more radiant complexion.

Ingredients

- 1 cup brown sugar

- 1/2 cup coconut oil

- 10 drops citrus essential oil (such as lemon, orange, or grapefruit)

Preparation Instructions:

- In a mixing bowl, combine the brown sugar and coconut oil.

- Add the citrus essential oil drops to the mixture and stir well to ensure even distribution.

Usage Instructions:

- Start by dampening your skin with warm water to prepare it for exfoliation.

- Take a small amount of the DIY Sugar Scrub and gently massage it onto your skin using circular motions, focusing on areas prone to dryness or roughness.

- Continue massaging for 2-3 minutes to allow the sugar granules to effectively exfoliate the skin.

- Rinse off the scrub with lukewarm water and pat your skin dry with a soft towel.

- Follow up with your favorite moisturizer to lock in hydration and keep your skin feeling soft and smooth.

Benefits for Different Skin Types:

- Exfoliation: The brown sugar granules provide gentle yet effective exfoliation, making this scrub suitable for all skin types, including sensitive skin.

- Hydration: Coconut oil is rich in moisturizing fatty acids that help hydrate and nourish the skin, leaving it feeling soft and supple.

- Invigoration: The citrus essential oils add a refreshing and invigorating scent to the scrub, awakening the senses and revitalizing the skin.

Storage and Shelf Life

Transfer any leftover DIY Sugar Scrub into an airtight container and store it in a cool, dry place. When stored properly, the scrub can last for up to several weeks.

6.3

Specialty Serums for Brightening and Firming

DIY Vitamin C Brightening Serum
Illuminate Your Skin

Experience the transformative power of our DIY Vitamin C Brightening Serum, a potent blend of vitamin C, hyaluronic acid, and botanical extracts designed to revitalize and rejuvenate your skin. This powerhouse serum targets uneven skin tone, hyperpigmentation, and signs of aging, leaving your complexion glowing with radiance and vitality.

Ingredients

- 1 teaspoon vitamin C powder (ascorbic acid)

- 1 tablespoon hyaluronic acid serum

- 1 teaspoon rosehip seed oil

- 5 drops botanical extracts (such as licorice extract or bearberry extract)

Preparation Instructions

- In a small mixing bowl, combine the vitamin C powder and hyaluronic acid serum.

- Stir the mixture until the vitamin C powder is fully dissolved.

- Add the rosehip seed oil and botanical extracts to the mixture, and stir well to ensure thorough incorporation.

Usage Instructions

- After cleansing and toning your skin, apply a few drops of the DIY Vitamin C Brightening Serum to your fingertips.

- Gently massage the serum onto your face and neck using upward, circular motions, avoiding the delicate eye area.

- Allow the serum to absorb fully into your skin before proceeding with your moisturizer or sunscreen.

- For best results, use the serum twice daily, in the morning and evening, as part of your skincare routine.

Benefits for Different Skin Types

- Brightening: Vitamin C is a powerful antioxidant that helps to brighten the skin and fade hyperpigmentation, making this serum ideal for those with dull or uneven skin tone.

- Hydration: Hyaluronic acid attracts and retains moisture in the skin, providing intense hydration and plumping fine lines and wrinkles, suitable for all skin types, including dry and dehydrated skin.

- Anti-aging: Rosehip seed oil is rich in vitamins A and C, as well as essential fatty acids, which promote collagen production and improve skin elasticity, making this serum beneficial for mature or aging skin.

Storage and Shelf Life

Store the DIY Vitamin C Brightening Serum in a dark, opaque container to protect it from light exposure, which can degrade the vitamin C over time. Keep the serum refrigerated to prolong its shelf life and maintain its efficacy. Discard any leftover serum after one to two weeks to ensure freshness and potency.

DIY Hyaluronic Acid Hydrating Serum
Quench Your Skin's Thirst

Indulge your skin with our DIY Hyaluronic Acid Hydrating Serum, a luxurious blend of hyaluronic acid, panthenol, and cucumber extract designed to hydrate, nourish, and rejuvenate your complexion. This lightweight yet deeply hydrating serum delivers intense moisture to parched skin, plumping fine lines and restoring suppleness for a radiant, youthful glow.

Ingredients

- 1 tablespoon hyaluronic acid serum

- 1 tablespoon panthenol (pro-vitamin B5)

- 1 tablespoon cucumber extract

Preparation Instructions

- In a small mixing bowl, combine the hyaluronic acid serum and panthenol.

- Stir the mixture until well blended and the ingredients are evenly distributed.

- Add the cucumber extract to the mixture and stir gently to incorporate.

Usage Instructions

- After cleansing and toning your skin, apply a few drops of the DIY Hyaluronic Acid Hydrating Serum to your fingertips.

- Gently massage the serum onto your face and neck using upward, circular motions, avoiding the eye area.

- Allow the serum to fully absorb into your skin before applying moisturizer or sunscreen.

- For optimal hydration, use the serum twice daily, in the morning and evening, as part of your skincare routine.

Benefits for Different Skin Types

- Hydration: Hyaluronic acid is a potent humectant that attracts and retains moisture in the skin, making this serum ideal for dry, dehydrated, or dull skin in need of intense hydration.

- Nourishment: Panthenol, or pro-vitamin B5, has soothing and moisturizing properties that help to strengthen the skin barrier and promote healing, making this serum suitable for sensitive or irritated skin.

- Rejuvenation: Cucumber extract is rich in antioxidants and vitamins, which help to rejuvenate and revitalize the skin, reducing the appearance of fine lines and improving overall skin tone and texture.

Storage and Shelf Life

Store the DIY Hyaluronic Acid Hydrating Serum in a dark, opaque container to protect it from light exposure, which can degrade the ingredients over time. Keep the serum refrigerated to prolong its shelf life and maintain its efficacy. Discard any leftover serum after one to two weeks to ensure freshness and potency.

Chapter 7

Advanced Techniques for Skincare Enthusiasts

Prepare to immerse yourself in formulations that marry high-quality ingredients with refined techniques, promising potent solutions for complex skin concerns and professional-grade results within the comforts of your own home.

Step into the realm of Anti-Aging Elixirs and Potions, where time stands still and beauty knows no bounds. Behold the Retinol Night Cream, a powerhouse blend of encapsulated retinol, peptides, and ceramides crafted to stimulate collagen production, diminish fine lines and wrinkles, and restore skin texture and elasticity. Meanwhile, the Coenzyme Q10 Serum emerges as a beacon of antioxidant protection, featuring coenzyme Q10, vitamin E, and squalane to combat oxidative damage, rejuvenate cells, and defy the signs of aging.

Indulge in the opulence of Luxurious Body Butters and Scrubs, where pampering meets perfection. Envelop your skin in the embrace of Whipped Shea Body Butter, a decadent fusion of shea butter, cocoa butter, and coconut oil designed to lavish dry skin with deep hydration, leaving it irresistibly soft, smooth, and supple. Then, invigorate your senses with the Coffee Scrub for Cellulite, a stimulating blend of coffee grounds, sugar, and grapefruit essential oil engineered to exfoliate, boost circulation, and minimize the appearance of cellulite.

Experience the radiance of DIY Sun Protection and After-Sun Care, where protection meets rejuvenation. Safeguard your skin with Homemade Sunscreen Lotion, a natural shield fortified with zinc oxide, red raspberry seed oil, and carrot seed oil, offering broad-spectrum UV protection while nourishing and moisturizing. And soothe sun-kissed skin with the Cooling Aloe Vera Gel, infused with aloe vera, cucumber extract, and lavender essential oil, working harmoniously to calm inflammation, reduce redness, and promote healing.

Each advanced-level recipe within this chapter is meticulously crafted, accompanied by detailed instructions, comprehensive ingredient lists, and invaluable tips for customization. With these formulations, skincare enthusiasts can luxuriate in the indulgence of professional-grade treatments tailored to their individual needs, all crafted with the finest natural ingredients.

7.1

Anti-Aging Elixirs and Potions

DIY Retinol Night Cream
Rejuvenate While You Sleep

Revitalize your skin with our DIY Retinol Night Cream, a potent anti-aging treatment infused with encapsulated retinol, peptides, and ceramides. This luxurious cream works overnight to stimulate collagen production, diminish fine lines and wrinkles, and enhance skin texture and elasticity, leaving you with a radiant and youthful complexion by morning.

Ingredients

- 1 tablespoon encapsulated retinol
- 1 tablespoon peptide complex
- 1 tablespoon ceramide concentrate

Preparation Instructions

- In a clean mixing bowl, combine the encapsulated retinol and peptide complex.
- Stir the mixture thoroughly until the ingredients are well blended.
- Add the ceramide concentrate to the mixture and continue stirring until fully incorporated.

Usage Instructions

- In the evening, after cleansing and toning your skin, apply a pea-sized amount of the DIY Retinol Night Cream to your face and neck.

- Gently massage the cream into your skin using upward, circular motions, ensuring even distribution.

- Allow the cream to absorb fully before applying any additional skincare products.

- Use the night cream consistently every evening as part of your nighttime skincare routine to maximize its anti-aging benefits.

Benefits for Different Skin Types

- Anti-Aging: Encapsulated retinol is a potent form of vitamin A that penetrates deeply into the skin to stimulate collagen production, reducing the appearance of fine lines and wrinkles. Peptides help to firm and lift the skin, while ceramides replenish lost moisture and strengthen the skin barrier, making this night cream suitable for mature or aging skin.

- Texture and Elasticity: The combination of retinol, peptides, and ceramides works synergistically to improve skin texture and elasticity, restoring smoothness and suppleness to the complexion. This night cream is ideal for those looking to address concerns such as roughness, uneven tone, and loss of firmness.

- Nourishment and Repair: Ceramides play a crucial role in maintaining the skin's natural moisture barrier and preventing moisture loss, making this night cream beneficial for dry or dehydrated skin in need of nourishment and repair.

Storage and Shelf Life

Store the DIY Retinol Night Cream in an airtight container to protect it from air and light exposure, which can degrade the potency of the ingredients. Keep the cream in a cool, dark place, such as a refrigerator, to prolong its shelf life and maintain its efficacy.

Use the night cream within one to two months of preparation to ensure freshness and effectiveness.

DIY Coenzyme Q10 Serum
Renew and Protect

Experience the power of antioxidants with our DIY Coenzyme Q10 Serum, a rejuvenating treatment enriched with coenzyme Q10, vitamin E, and squalane. This potent serum defends against oxidative stress, supports cellular renewal, and diminishes signs of aging, leaving your skin with a radiant and youthful glow.

Ingredients

- 1 teaspoon coenzyme Q10 powder

- 1 tablespoon vitamin E oil

- 2 tablespoons squalane oil

Preparation Instructions:

- In a clean mixing bowl, combine the coenzyme Q10 powder and vitamin E oil.

- Stir the mixture thoroughly until the coenzyme Q10 is fully dissolved in the oil.

- Add the squalane oil to the mixture and continue stirring until all ingredients are well combined.

Usage Instructions

- After cleansing and toning your skin, apply a few drops of the DIY Coenzyme Q10 Serum to your face and neck.

- Gently massage the serum into your skin using upward, circular motions until fully absorbed.

- Follow with your favorite moisturizer or sunscreen as needed.

- Use the serum twice daily, morning and evening, as part of your skincare routine for optimal results.

Benefits for Different Skin Types

- Antioxidant Protection: Coenzyme Q10 and vitamin E are powerful antioxidants that help neutralize free radicals and protect the skin from environmental damage, making this serum ideal for all skin types, especially those exposed to pollution or UV radiation.

- Cell Renewal: Coenzyme Q10 supports cellular energy production and metabolism, promoting cell renewal and regeneration. Vitamin E further enhances this process by nourishing and repairing damaged skin cells, resulting in a smoother and more youthful complexion.

- Anti-Aging: Squalane oil is deeply hydrating and emollient, helping to reduce the appearance of fine lines and wrinkles while improving skin elasticity and firmness. Combined with coenzyme Q10 and vitamin E, this serum effectively diminishes signs of aging and restores a youthful radiance to the skin.

Storage and Shelf Life

Store the DIY Coenzyme Q10 Serum in a dark, glass dropper bottle to protect it from light exposure, which can degrade the potency of the ingredients. Keep the serum in a cool, dry place away from direct sunlight to maintain its efficacy. Use the serum within one to two months of preparation to ensure freshness and effectiveness.

7.2

Luxurious Body Butters and Scrubs

DIY Whipped Shea Body Butter
Indulge Your Skin

Pamper your skin with our luxurious DIY Whipped Shea Body Butter, a sumptuous blend of shea butter, cocoa butter, and coconut oil. This rich and creamy body butter deeply nourishes and hydrates dry skin, leaving it irresistibly soft, smooth, and supple. Treat yourself to the ultimate indulgence and discover the transformative power of natural ingredients.

Ingredients

- 1/2 cup shea butter

- 1/4 cup cocoa butter

- 1/4 cup coconut oil

- Optional: a few drops of your favorite essential oil for fragrance (such as lavender, rose, or citrus)

Preparation Instructions

- In a heat-safe bowl, combine the shea butter, cocoa butter, and coconut oil.

- Gently melt the ingredients together using a double boiler or microwave, stirring occasionally until fully melted.

- Once melted, remove the bowl from the heat and let the mixture cool for a few minutes.

- If using essential oils for fragrance, add a few drops to the mixture and stir well to combine.

- Place the bowl in the refrigerator to chill for about 15-20 minutes, or until the mixture begins to solidify around the edges.

• Once the edges start to harden, remove the bowl from the refrigerator and use a hand mixer or stand mixer to whip the mixture until light and fluffy.

• Continue whipping for 5-10 minutes, or until the body butter reaches a creamy, whipped consistency.

• Transfer the whipped body butter to a clean, airtight jar or container for storage.

Usage Instructions

• Scoop a small amount of the DIY Whipped Shea Body Butter into your hands.

• Gently massage the body butter onto clean, dry skin, focusing on areas prone to dryness such as elbows, knees, and heels.

• Allow the body butter to absorb fully into the skin before dressing.

• Use daily as part of your skincare routine to keep your skin soft, smooth, and hydrated.

Benefits for Different Skin Types

• Dry Skin: Shea butter, cocoa butter, and coconut oil are all deeply hydrating and emollient, making this body butter perfect for those with dry skin. These rich ingredients penetrate deeply into the skin, providing intense moisture and nourishment to leave skin feeling soft and supple.

• Sensitive Skin: The natural ingredients in this body butter are gentle and soothing, making it suitable for sensitive skin types. Shea butter and cocoa butter have anti-inflammatory properties that help calm irritation and redness, while coconut oil is non-comedogenic and unlikely to cause breakouts.

Storage and Shelf Life:

Store the DIY Whipped Shea Body Butter in a cool, dry place away from direct sunlight to prevent melting. The body butter should last for several months if stored properly. If you notice any changes in texture or smell, discard the product and make a fresh batch.

DIY Coffee Scrub for Cellulite
Awaken Your Skin

Revitalize your skin and invigorate your senses with our DIY Coffee Scrub for Cellulite, a stimulating blend of coffee grounds, sugar, and grapefruit essential oil. This rejuvenating body scrub gently exfoliates, improves circulation, and helps reduce the appearance of cellulite, leaving your skin smooth, firm, and radiant. Say goodbye to dull, uneven skin and awaken your body to a renewed sense of vitality and confidence.

Ingredients

- 1/2 cup coffee grounds

- 1/2 cup granulated sugar

- 1/4 cup coconut oil (or any carrier oil of your choice)

- 10-15 drops grapefruit essential oil

Preparation Instructions:

- In a mixing bowl, combine the coffee grounds and granulated sugar.

- Melt the coconut oil in a microwave-safe bowl or double boiler until it becomes liquid.

- Pour the melted coconut oil over the coffee grounds and sugar mixture.

- Add 10-15 drops of grapefruit essential oil to the bowl and stir well to combine all the ingredients thoroughly.

- Transfer the mixture to a clean, airtight jar or container for storage.

Usage Instructions

- Begin by wetting your skin with warm water to soften it.

- Take a generous amount of the DIY Coffee Scrub and massage it onto your skin using circular motions, focusing on areas prone to cellulite such as thighs, buttocks, and hips.

- Continue massaging for 5-10 minutes to allow the caffeine and exfoliating particles to stimulate circulation and promote lymphatic drainage.

- Rinse off the scrub with warm water and pat your skin dry with a towel.

- Follow up with a hydrating body lotion or oil to lock in moisture and further nourish your skin.

Benefits for Different Skin Types

- All Skin Types: The gentle exfoliation provided by the coffee grounds and sugar helps slough away dead skin cells, revealing smoother, more radiant skin underneath. The caffeine in coffee grounds stimulates blood flow and helps reduce the appearance of cellulite, making this scrub suitable for all skin types.

- Dull, Uneven Skin: The invigorating scent of grapefruit essential oil helps uplift your mood and awaken your senses, while its astringent properties help tone and tighten the skin, leaving it looking firmer and more youthful.

Storage and Shelf Life

Store the DIY Coffee Scrub in a cool, dry place away from direct sunlight. It should last for several weeks if stored properly. If you notice any changes in texture or smell, discard the scrub and make a fresh batch.

7.3

DIY Sun Protection and After-Sun Care

Homemade Sunscreen Lotion
Protect and Nourish Your Skin

Shield your skin naturally with our Sunscreen Lotion, a homemade blend crafted with zinc oxide, red raspberry seed oil, carrot seed oil, and - if you want to add sweetness and smoothness - coconut oil to provide broad-spectrum UV protection while nourishing and moisturizing the skin.

Ingredients

- 1/4 cup zinc oxide

- 2 tablespoons red raspberry seed oil

- 1 tablespoon carrot seed oil

- Optional: 1 tablespoon coconut oil

Preparation Instructions

- In a clean bowl, combine 1/4 cup of zinc oxide with 2 tablespoons of red raspberry seed oil, 1 tablespoon of carrot seed oil, and 1 tablespoon of coconut oil.

- Mix the ingredients thoroughly until well incorporated, ensuring the zinc oxide is evenly distributed.

- Transfer the mixture to an airtight container or squeeze bottle for convenient application.

Usage Instructions

- Before sun exposure, apply a generous amount of the Homemade Sunscreen Lotion to clean, dry skin.

- Massage the lotion evenly onto the skin until fully absorbed, focusing on areas prone to sun exposure.

- Reapply every two hours or after swimming or sweating to maintain effective protection.

Benefits for Different Skin Types

- Broad-Spectrum Protection: Zinc oxide provides broad-spectrum UV protection, shielding the skin from both UVA and UVB rays.

- Nourishing: Red raspberry seed oil, carrot seed oil, and coconut oil nourish and moisturize the skin, preventing dryness and promoting a healthy complexion.

- Natural Ingredients: This homemade sunscreen lotion is free from synthetic chemicals and harsh additives, making it suitable for all skin types, including sensitive skin.

Storage and Shelf Life

Store the Homemade Sunscreen Lotion in a cool, dry place away from direct sunlight. It can typically be kept for up to three to six months. For best results, use within a few months of preparation.

DIY Aloe Vera Gel for Sunburn Relief
Soothe Your Skin

Relieve sunburned skin and restore its natural balance with our DIY Cooling Aloe Vera Gel. This soothing after-sun treatment is enriched with the healing properties of aloe vera, cucumber extract, and lavender essential oil to calm irritation, reduce inflammation, and promote skin healing. Whether you've spent a little too much time under the sun or simply want to pamper your skin after exposure, this cooling gel will provide instant relief and nourishment.

Ingredients

- 1/4 cup pure aloe vera gel

- 2 tablespoons cucumber extract or cucumber juice

- 5-7 drops lavender essential oil

Preparation Instructions

- In a small bowl, combine the pure aloe vera gel and cucumber extract.

- Add 5-7 drops of lavender essential oil to the mixture and stir well to incorporate.

- Transfer the mixture to a clean, airtight container for storage.

Usage Instructions

- After spending time in the sun, gently cleanse your skin with a mild, non-drying cleanser.

- Apply a generous amount of the DIY Cooling Aloe Vera Gel to the affected areas of your skin, such as sunburned or irritated areas.

- Gently massage the gel into your skin until it is fully absorbed.

- Allow the gel to remain on your skin and reapply as needed for continuous relief and hydration.

Benefits for Different Skin Types

- Sunburned or Irritated Skin: Aloe vera is renowned for its soothing and healing properties, making it ideal for calming sunburned or irritated skin. Cucumber extract provides additional hydration and cooling relief, while lavender essential oil helps reduce inflammation and promote skin regeneration.

- Sensitive or Reactive Skin: The gentle, non-irritating formula of this DIY Cooling Aloe Vera Gel makes it suitable for all skin types, including sensitive or reactive skin. It provides instant relief from sunburn, redness, and discomfort without causing further irritation.

Storage and Shelf Life

Store the DIY Cooling Aloe Vera Gel in a cool, dry place away from direct sunlight. It should last for several weeks if stored properly. If you notice any changes in texture or smell, discard the gel and make a fresh batch.

Troubleshooting and Customization

The path of DIY skincare, while exciting, can sometimes present unexpected detours. This chapter equips you to navigate these challenges with confidence. We'll explore common pitfalls encountered during formulation, like frustrating emulsion breakage or ingredient separation. Fear not! We'll provide solutions – adjusting oil-to-water ratios, incorporating stabilizing emulsifiers, and ensuring proper mixing techniques.

But the true beauty of DIY skincare lies in customization. This chapter empowers you to tailor your creations to your unique skin's story. Whether you battle oily skin and yearn for lightweight textures, or your dry skin craves rich emollients, we'll provide guidelines for adapting recipes to perfectly suit your needs.

Going beyond basic skin types, we'll delve into targeting specific concerns. Acne, aging, hyperpigmentation, sensitivity – these are all battles many fight. We'll explore how to customize formulations through strategic ingredient selection, allowing you to craft solutions that address your personal struggles.

Remember, your skin's needs don't stay constant. Winter's dryness requires different attention than summer's sun exposure. This chapter offers tips for modifying your formulations seasonally, adjusting hydration levels, incorporating sun protection, and utilizing appropriate botanicals to optimize your skincare routine year-round.

Finally, we emphasize the importance of quality control. Learn how to conduct sensory evaluations, ensuring your creations meet your desired feel and scent. Don't let your hard work go to waste – stability testing will help evaluate shelf life and efficacy under various storage conditions. Most importantly, safety comes first. We'll discuss patch testing, a crucial step to assess potential allergic reactions to new ingredients, minimizing risks before widespread use

8.1

Understanding Formulation Challenges and Solutions

Emulsion Instability
Applying Troubleshooting Strategies

Emulsion instability in skincare formulation often arises due to several interrelated factors, each contributing to the breakdown of the oil and water phases. One common issue is an imbalance in the oil-to-water ratio, where an excessive amount of one phase overwhelms the other, leading to phase separation or creaming. For example, in a water-in-oil (W/O) emulsion, if the oil phase dominates, the water droplets may coalesce and rise to the surface, resulting in a greasy or separated product.

To address this imbalance, formulators may adjust the oil-to-water ratio by increasing the water phase or reducing the oil phase, depending on the desired product characteristics. For instance, in a lightweight lotion, increasing the water content while maintaining adequate emulsification can enhance product spreadability and absorption, reducing the risk of emulsion instability.

Another crucial factor in stabilizing emulsions is the selection and incorporation of suitable emulsifiers. Emulsifiers work by lowering the interfacial tension between oil and water phases, preventing them from separating. Examples of effective emulsifiers include lecithin, polysorbates, and glyceryl stearate. By choosing emulsifiers with compatible hydrophilic-lipophilic balance (HLB) values and incorporating them at appropriate concentrations, formulators can improve emulsion stability and prevent phase separation.

Practical examples illustrate how troubleshooting strategies are applied in skincare formulation. Suppose a formulator encounters phase separation in a moisturizing cream containing water, oils, and emulsifiers. To address this issue, they may experiment with adjusting the oil-to-water ratio by increasing the water phase and incorporating a higher concentration of emulsifiers with suitable

HLB values. By optimizing these variables and conducting stability tests, the formulator can achieve a stable emulsion with uniform texture and appearance.

Furthermore, optimizing mixing techniques is essential for achieving homogeneity and uniform dispersion of ingredients in the emulsion. High-shear mixing methods, such as high-speed blending or homogenization, help break down particle aggregates and ensure thorough emulsification. By controlling mixing speed, duration, and temperature, formulators can promote emulsion stability and prevent issues like phase separation or creaming.

Case studies provide valuable insights into real-world applications of troubleshooting strategies. For instance, a formulator may encounter emulsion instability in a facial serum containing water, botanical oils, and natural emulsifiers. By systematically adjusting formulation parameters, such as oil-to-water ratio, emulsifier type and concentration, and mixing techniques, the formulator can identify the root cause of instability and implement effective solutions to achieve a stable, high-quality product.

Addressing emulsion instability in skincare formulation requires a comprehensive understanding of the underlying factors and systematic troubleshooting approaches. By adjusting formulation parameters, incorporating suitable emulsifiers, optimizing mixing techniques, and drawing insights from practical examples and case studies, formulators can overcome challenges and achieve stable emulsions that meet the desired performance and aesthetic requirements.

Ingredient Separation
Strategies for Product Integrity

Ingredient separation is a common issue encountered in skincare formulations, where the components fail to remain uniformly dispersed, resulting in visible layers or clumps. This phenomenon can occur due to various factors such as differences in ingredient polarity, incompatibilities between components, inadequate emulsification, or insufficient viscosity. To effectively address and prevent ingredient separation, skincare formulators employ a range of techniques and strategies aimed at enhancing stability and ensuring product integrity.

Proper emulsification techniques play a crucial role in preventing ingredient separation by facilitating the uniform dispersion of immiscible phases, such as oil and water. High-shear mixing methods, such as homogenization or high-speed blending, are commonly employed to break down and disperse the ingredients evenly, thereby minimizing the risk of phase separation.

Ensuring compatibility between ingredients is essential to prevent separation. Formulators must consider factors such as the polarity, solubility, and chemical reactivity of each component to avoid incompatibilities that could lead to phase separation. Compatibility testing, which involves combining ingredients and observing for signs of instability, helps identify suitable combinations and mitigate the risk of separation.

The selection and incorporation of appropriate thickeners and stabilizers are key strategies for preventing ingredient separation in skincare formulations. Thickeners, such as gums (e.g., xanthan gum, guar gum) or polymers (e.g., carbomer), increase the viscosity of the formulation, improving stability and reducing the likelihood of phase separation. Stabilizers, such as surfactants or emulsifiers, help maintain the integrity of the emulsion by preventing the coalescence or aggregation of dispersed phases.

Optimizing formulation parameters, including the concentration of emulsifiers, pH level, and viscosity modifiers, can significantly contribute to stability and prevent separation. Fine-tuning these parameters based on compatibility testing and performance evaluations allows formulators to achieve the desired texture, appearance, and stability of the final product.

Regular testing and quality control measures are essential for identifying and addressing potential issues related to ingredient separation. Stability studies, accelerated aging tests, and compatibility assessments help assess the long-term stability and performance of the formulation under various conditions, ensuring that the product remains stable and uniform throughout its shelf life.

Practical examples and case studies can provide valuable insights into overcoming ingredient separation challenges. For instance, adjusting the emulsifier system, optimizing the viscosity profile, or incorporating additional stabilizers may help stabilize formulations and prevent separation. By documenting these experiences and lessons learned, formulators can refine their techniques and develop more robust formulations in the future.

Preventing ingredient separation in skincare formulations requires a comprehensive understanding of the underlying factors and effective implementation of preventive strategies. By employing proper emulsification techniques, ensuring ingredient compatibility, utilizing appropriate thickeners and stabilizers, optimizing formulation parameters, and conducting rigorous testing and quality control measures, formulators can enhance stability and maintain product integrity, resulting in high-quality and reliable skincare products.

Ingredients, Thickeners and Stabilizers
How to Prevent Ingredient Separation

Texture and consistency are crucial aspects of skincare products, influencing their feel, application, and effectiveness. However, achieving the desired texture and consistency can be challenging due to various factors such as ingredient interactions, processing methods, and formulation techniques. To address texture and consistency issues effectively, skincare formulators employ a range of techniques and strategies aimed at optimizing ingredient proportions, incorporating texture-modifying agents, and refining formulation methods.

Adjusting ingredient proportions is a fundamental strategy for achieving the desired texture and consistency in skincare formulations. By carefully balancing the ratios of key ingredients such as oils, emulsifiers, thickeners, and water, formulators can tailor the product's texture to meet specific requirements. For example, increasing the concentration of oils or butters can result in a richer, more emollient texture, while adjusting the amount of water or humectants can influence the product's viscosity and hydration level.

Incorporating texture-modifying agents is another effective approach for addressing texture and consistency issues in skincare products. Texture-modifying agents, such as gelling agents, rheology modifiers, and film formers, can alter the physical properties of the formulation to achieve the desired texture, thickness, or spreadability. For instance, adding natural gums like xanthan gum or carrageenan can thicken the product and improve its stability, while silicone-based polymers can impart a smooth, silky feel to the formulation.

Optimizing formulation methods is essential for ensuring consistent texture and performance in skincare products. Formulators may experiment with different mixing techniques, processing temperatures, and homogenization methods to achieve the desired emulsion stability and particle size distribution. High-shear mixing, sonication, and microfluidization are commonly used methods for dispersing and blending ingredients to create homogeneous formulations with uniform texture and consistency.

Conducting thorough performance evaluations and sensory assessments is critical for identifying and addressing texture and consistency issues in skincare products. Formulators may utilize techniques such as texture analysis, rheological testing, and consumer panel evaluations to assess parameters such as viscosity, spreadability, tackiness, and skin feel. By soliciting feedback from consumers and conducting objective measurements, formulators can refine the formulation to meet desired texture and consistency standards.

Practical examples and case studies can provide valuable insights into addressing texture and consistency issues in skincare formulations. For instance, adjusting the pH level, incorporating co-solvents or co-emulsifiers, or optimizing the processing conditions may help improve the product's texture and stability. By documenting these experiences and lessons learned, formulators can refine their techniques and develop more aesthetically pleasing and user-friendly skincare products in the future.

In conclusion, achieving the desired texture and consistency in skincare products requires a combination of careful ingredient selection, formulation optimization, and performance testing. By ad-

8.2

Tailoring Recipes
to Address Individual Needs

Formulations to Suit Every Skin Type
Guidelines for Customization

Customizing skincare formulations for specific skin types is a crucial aspect of creating effective and targeted skincare products. By adjusting skincare recipes to accommodate different skin types, formulators can ensure that their products address the unique needs and concerns of each individual. Here are some guidelines for customizing formulations based on specific skin types:

Understanding the Characteristics: Before customizing formulations, it's essential to have a thorough understanding of the characteristics of different skin types. Common skin types include oily, dry, combination, and sensitive. Oily skin tends to produce excess sebum and is prone to acne, while dry skin lacks moisture and may feel tight or rough.

Incorporating Lightweight Ingredients for Oily Skin: For oily skin types, it's important to incorporate lightweight and non-comedogenic ingredients that won't clog pores or exacerbate oiliness. Ingredients such as hyaluronic acid, niacinamide, and lightweight oils like jojoba or grapeseed oil can help hydrate the skin without adding excess shine.

Adding Rich Emollients for Dry Skin: Conversely, dry skin requires rich emollients and humectants to replenish moisture and restore the skin's natural barrier. Ingredients such as shea butter, cocoa butter, and oils like avocado or almond oil provide deep hydration and nourishment for dry skin, helping to alleviate tightness and flakiness.

Balancing Hydration for Combination Skin: Combination skin presents a unique challenge, as it requires balancing hydration without exacerbating oiliness in certain areas. Formulations for combination skin should include a combination of lightweight hydrators for oily areas and richer emollients for dry patches. Ingredients like hyaluronic acid, glycerin, and lightweight oils can help balance hydration levels in combination skin.

Choosing Gentle Formulations for Sensitive Skin: Sensitive skin requires gentle formulations free from harsh or irritating ingredients. Fragrance-free, hypoallergenic, and non-comedogenic products are ideal for sensitive skin types. Ingredients like chamomile extract, aloe vera, and colloidal oatmeal can help soothe and calm sensitive skin while providing hydration and nourishment.

Adjusting Active Ingredients Based on Skin Concerns: In addition to selecting appropriate base ingredients, formulators can adjust the concentration of active ingredients based on specific skin concerns. For example, acne-prone skin may benefit from higher concentrations of salicylic acid or tea tree oil, while anti-aging formulations may include higher levels of retinol or vitamin C for mature skin.

Maintaining pH Balance: Maintaining the pH balance of skincare formulations is crucial for ensuring compatibility with the skin's natural pH level. Formulators should choose ingredients and adjust formulations to maintain a slightly acidic pH, typically around 4.5 to 5.5, which helps support the skin's protective acid mantle.

Addressing Targeted Concerns: Customizing formulations for specific skin concerns allows formulators to address targeted issues such as acne, hyperpigmentation, or fine lines. Incorporating ingredients like alpha hydroxy acids (AHAs), beta hydroxy acids (BHAs), or botanical extracts can help target specific skin concerns while maintaining overall skin health.

Conducting Patch Testing: Before introducing customized formulations to clients or customers, it's essential to conduct patch testing to ensure compatibility and minimize the risk of adverse reactions. Patch testing involves applying a small amount of product to a discreet area of skin and monitoring for any signs of irritation or sensitivity over 24 to 48 hours.

Monitoring and Adjusting Formulations: Skincare formulations may need to be adjusted over time based on feedback from users and changes in environmental factors. Formulators should monitor the performance and efficacy of their products and be prepared to make adjustments as needed to optimize results.

Consulting with Professionals: For complex skincare concerns or formulations, consulting with skincare professionals such as dermatologists or cosmetic chemists can provide valuable insights and guidance. Professionals can help assess individual skin needs and recommend appropriate ingredients and formulations to achieve desired results.

Customizing skincare formulations for specific skin types is essential for creating effective and targeted products that address the unique needs and concerns of each individual. By understanding the characteristics of different skin types and following these guidelines, formulators can create skincare products that promote overall skin health and vitality.

Formulations to Target Skin Concerns
Crafting Personalized Solutions

Customizing skincare formulations to tackle specific skin concerns involves a thoughtful process that merges ingredient expertise with tailored formulation techniques. This approach empowers skincare enthusiasts to create personalized solutions that cater to their unique skin needs. Let's delve into how this is achieved.

Firstly, it's vital to grasp the root causes behind common skin issues like acne, aging signs, hyperpigmentation, and sensitivity. For instance, acne can stem from factors like excess oil production and bacterial growth, while aging skin often reflects collagen depletion and environmental damage.

Incorporating active ingredients is a pivotal step in addressing these concerns effectively. Ingredients such as salicylic acid, retinoids, and antioxidants play key roles in combating specific issues. Salicylic acid unclogs pores and reduces inflammation in acne-prone skin, while retinoids stimulate collagen synthesis to minimize fine lines and wrinkles.

To tailor formulations to individual needs, formulators adjust ingredient concentrations and blend synergistic combinations. Higher concentrations of active ingredients in serums and treatments offer targeted solutions. However, it's essential to strike a balance by including soothing and hydrating agents like aloe vera and chamomile extract to prevent irritation, especially in formulations for sensitive skin.

Customization extends beyond active ingredients to texture, scent, and potency. Lightweight, mattifying textures suit oily skin, while rich, emollient formulations provide nourishment for dry skin. Additionally, incorporating preventative measures such as sunscreen and antioxidants safeguards skin health and prevents future issues.

Remaining informed about emerging ingredients is crucial. Niacinamide, hyaluronic acid, and bakuchiol are examples of versatile ingredients that offer multifaceted benefits for various skin concerns. Seeking advice from skincare professionals, such as dermatologists or estheticians, ensures personalized recommendations tailored to individual needs.

Before introducing new formulations, patch testing is essential to assess compatibility and minimize the risk of adverse reactions. This involves applying a small amount of product to a discreet area of skin and monitoring for any signs of irritation.

Continuous monitoring and adjustment of formulations based on user feedback and emerging research are necessary for optimizing results. This iterative process ensures that skincare products remain effective and relevant to evolving skin needs.

In summary, customizing skincare formulations involves understanding skin concerns, incorporating effective ingredients, and tailoring formulations to individual preferences. By adopting this approach, skincare enthusiasts can create personalized solutions that promote healthier, more radiant skin.

Seasonal Skincare Solutions
Adapting Your Routine for Changing Weather

As the seasons transition, our skincare needs evolve alongside the shifting environmental conditions. Just as we update our wardrobe with the changing weather, it's essential to adjust our skincare routine to ensure our skin stays healthy and radiant throughout the year. In this column, we'll explore some simple yet effective strategies for adapting your skincare formulations to meet the demands of each season.

Winter Wonder Moisture

As temperatures drop and humidity levels plummet, our skin tends to become drier and more prone to irritation. Combat winter woes with hydration-rich formulations that provide a nourishing barrier against harsh weather conditions. Look for moisturizers and serums infused with ingredients like hyaluronic acid, shea butter, and ceramides to replenish lost moisture and protect your skin from winter's chill.

Spring into Soothing Sensations

With the arrival of spring comes a renewed focus on calming and soothing skincare solutions. After months of exposure to cold winds and indoor heating, our skin may be in need of some TLC.

Incorporate botanical extracts like aloe vera, chamomile, and cucumber into your skincare routine to soothe inflammation, reduce redness, and restore balance to your complexion.

Summer Sun Protection

As the sun shines brighter and temperatures soar, it's crucial to ramp up your sun protection game. Swap out your regular moisturizer for one that contains SPF and reapply throughout the day, especially if you're spending time outdoors. Additionally, consider adding antioxidant-rich serums and lightweight hydrating mists to your routine to combat the damaging effects of UV radiation and keep your skin feeling refreshed and rejuvenated.

Fall for Antioxidant-Rich Formulations

As the leaves change color and the air becomes crisper, it's time to embrace antioxidant-rich skincare formulations. Ingredients like vitamin C, green tea extract, and niacinamide can help protect your skin from environmental aggressors, reduce the appearance of fine lines and wrinkles, and promote a radiant complexion. Incorporate these powerhouse ingredients into your fall skincare routine to keep your skin looking youthful and vibrant as the seasons change.

Listen to Your Skin

While seasonal skincare guidelines provide a helpful framework, it's essential to listen to your skin's unique needs and adjust your routine accordingly. Pay attention to how your skin responds to changes in weather and environmental factors, and tailor your skincare regimen to address any concerns that arise. By tuning into your skin's signals and adapting your routine as needed, you can ensure that your complexion stays healthy and glowing all year long.

Adapting your skincare routine to the changing seasons is a simple yet effective way to keep your skin looking and feeling its best year-round. By incorporating hydrating ingredients in the winter, soothing botanicals in the spring, sun protection in the summer, and antioxidants in the fall, you can address seasonal skincare concerns and maintain a radiant complexion no matter what the weather brings. So, embrace the beauty of each season and treat your skin to the care it deserves!

8.3

Product Testing and Quality Control

Unlocking the Senses
The Power of Sensory Evaluation in Skincare

Sensory evaluation is a critical aspect of skincare product development, enabling formulators to meticulously assess various sensory attributes such as texture, scent, and overall feel. This process is essential for ensuring that skincare products not only deliver effective results but also provide a delightful sensory experience for the user.

One of the key elements evaluated during sensory testing is the texture of the product. Skincare enthusiasts have diverse preferences when it comes to texture – some may prefer lightweight, fast-absorbing formulations, while others may favor richer, more nourishing textures. For example, a lightweight gel moisturizer may be preferred during hot summer months for its refreshing feel, while a luxurious cream may be more suitable for dry winter skin in need of intense hydration.

In addition to texture, scent plays a crucial role in determining the overall appeal of skincare products. Fragrance can evoke emotions, trigger memories, and create a sense of luxury and indulgence. However, it's essential to strike the right balance – the scent should be pleasant and subtle, enhancing the user experience without overwhelming the senses. For instance, a gentle floral or citrus scent may be preferred in a daytime moisturizer, while a soothing lavender scent may be more suitable for a night cream aimed at promoting relaxation and sleep.

The overall feel of a skincare product on the skin is another aspect evaluated during sensory testing. Factors such as smoothness, hydration, and absorption rate contribute to the user's perception of the product's efficacy and comfort. Sensory evaluation helps formulators fine-tune these attributes to ensure optimal performance and user satisfaction. For example, a serum formulated with hyaluronic acid and glycerin may be designed to provide an instant boost of hydration while leaving the skin feeling silky-smooth and non-greasy.

Conducting sensory tests involves gathering feedback from a diverse group of individuals representing the target demographic. Participants are asked to use the product and provide detailed feedback on various sensory aspects, including texture, scent, and skin feel. This feedback is invaluable for identifying areas of improvement and refining the formulation accordingly. For instance, a panel of testers may be asked to rate a moisturizer on attributes such as spreadability, absorbency, and residual tackiness.

One of the challenges of sensory evaluation is ensuring consistency and reliability in the testing process. Formulators must establish standardized testing protocols and criteria to ensure accurate and reproducible results. This may involve conducting blind tests, using controlled environments, and employing trained sensory panelists. For example, testers may be instructed to apply the product to clean, dry skin and evaluate its sensory attributes at various intervals over a specified period.

Advancements in technology have also facilitated sensory evaluation in skincare product development. For example, instrumental methods such as texture analyzers and olfactometers can provide objective measurements of texture and scent, complementing traditional sensory testing methods. These tools help formulators quantify sensory attributes and identify subtle changes in product performance.

Ultimately, the goal of sensory evaluation is to create skincare products that not only deliver tangible benefits for the skin but also provide a delightful sensorial experience. By paying attention to details such as texture, scent, and overall feel, formulators can create products that resonate with consumers on a deeper level. For example, a luxurious facial oil may be formulated with a silky-smooth texture and a delicate floral scent to evoke feelings of indulgence and self-care during application.

In conclusion, sensory evaluation plays a crucial role in the development of skincare products, allowing formulators to fine-tune various sensory attributes to meet the preferences of their target audience. By leveraging feedback from sensory testing, skincare brands can create products that not only deliver effective results but also provide a luxurious and enjoyable experience for users.

Stability Testing: Performing stability tests to evaluate the shelf life and efficacy of skincare formulations under various storage conditions, identifying potential issues and making necessary adjustments.

Stability Testing
Ensuring the Integrity of DIY Skincare

Stability testing is an essential step in the development of any skincare product, including those formulated at home. This process evaluates how a product performs over time under various environmental conditions such as temperature, humidity, and light exposure. The primary goal is to ensure the product maintains its efficacy, texture, color, and safety throughout its intended shelf life.

Importance of Stability Testing for DIY Products

While stability testing may seem unnecessary for DIY skincare enthusiasts, it plays a crucial role in guaranteeing the safety and effectiveness of your homemade creations over time. Natural ingredients, while gentle and beneficial, can be more susceptible to variation and quicker degradation compared to synthetic components. Stability testing helps identify potential issues like bacterial growth, phase separation, or changes in scent and texture, which could indicate the product is no longer suitable for use.

Basic Stability Testing Methods for Home Use

Performing basic stability testing at home doesn't require a sophisticated laboratory setup. Transforming your kitchen or bathroom into a mini-lab is simpler than it sounds. Here are some simple methods you can implement:

- *Temperature Variation Testing*: Store samples of your product at different temperatures – room temperature, refrigerated, and a warm environment (near a heater or sunny window). Observe any changes in texture, smell, or color over a period of one to three months.

- *Container Testing*: Different containers can interact with your product in varying ways. Test your product in various containers made of glass, plastic, and metal to observe any interactions or degradation.

- *Light Exposure Testing*: Expose the product to different lighting conditions – direct sunlight, ambient light, and darkness. Natural ingredients are often sensitive to light, which can degrade some essential oils and botanical extracts.

Recording Observations

- Maintain a detailed log to record your observations:

- Date of formulation and each subsequent evaluation

- Descriptions of any changes in color, texture, scent, and separation

- Presence of mold or unusual microbial growth

- Formulation Adjustments Based on Observations

Based on your observations, you may need to modify your formulation:

- *Preservatives*: If you notice signs of microbial growth, consider incorporating a natural preservative such as Grapefruit Seed Extract or Vitamin E.

- *Antioxidants*: To combat rancidity and color changes, antioxidants like Green Tea Extract or Rosemary Oil Extract can be added.

- *Emulsifiers and Stabilizers*: If your product separates, consider incorporating a natural emulsifier or stabilizer like xanthan gum or lecithin.

Advanced Considerations for Stability Testing

For those who wish to take their testing further, here are some additional considerations:

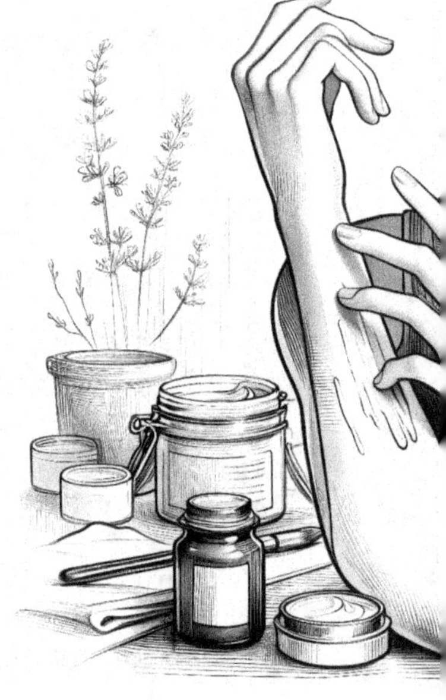

- *pH Testing Kits*: Maintaining the optimal pH level for skin (typically between 4.5 and 5.5) is crucial for product stability and preventing irritation. A pH testing kit can help ensure your formulation remains within this ideal range.

- *Microbial Testing Kits*: These kits are available for home use and can provide assurance that your product is free from harmful bacteria and fungi.

While stability testing at home cannot replicate the capabilities of a professional laboratory, it offers valuable insight into the performance of your DIY skincare products over time. This process is invaluable for crafting effective, safe, and high-quality natural skincare products. Through careful observation and adjustments based on your testing, you can ensure that your homemade creations are both enjoyable and beneficial for your skin.

Patch Testing
Shielding Skin Through Precautionary Measures

Patch testing is a fundamental step in skincare safety, serving as a precautionary measure to assess the skin's reaction to new ingredients. This process involves applying a small amount of product to a discreet area of skin and monitoring for any signs of allergic reactions or sensitivities. By conducting patch tests, individuals can minimize the risk of adverse reactions when using skincare products on a larger scale.

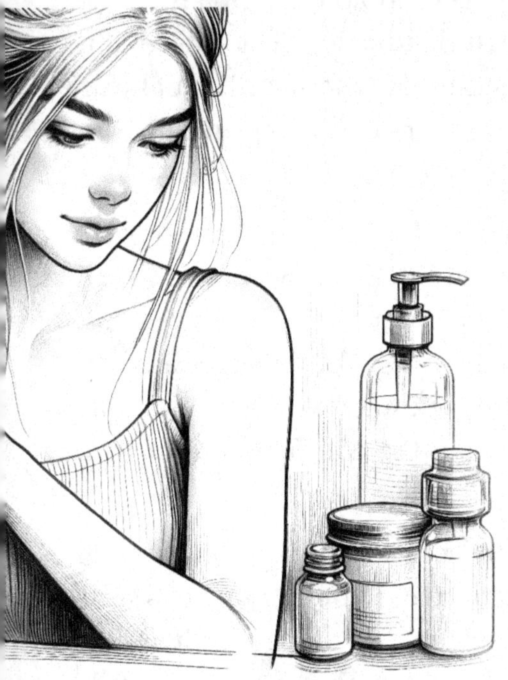

The primary purpose of patch testing is to identify potential allergens or irritants before widespread application to the skin. This is particularly important for individuals with sensitive skin or a history of allergies, as they may be more prone to adverse reactions. Patch testing allows them to evaluate the compatibility of a new product with their skin and make informed decisions about its suitability for regular use.

The process of patch testing is relatively straightforward. A small amount of the product is applied to a clean, dry area of skin, such as the inner forearm or behind the ear. The area is then covered with a patch or adhesive bandage to prevent the product from being rubbed off or coming into contact with other surfaces. After 24 to 48 hours, the patch is removed, and the skin is examined for any signs of redness, itching, swelling, or other adverse reactions.

It's essential to conduct patch tests for each new product or ingredient, as sensitivities can vary depending on the formulation. Even if a product is labeled as "natural" or "gentle," it can still cause reactions in some individuals. Patch testing provides a proactive approach to skincare safety, allowing users to identify potential allergens or irritants before they cause significant discomfort or damage to the skin.

Patch testing is especially crucial when introducing products with potent active ingredients, such as retinoids or alpha hydroxy acids, which can cause irritation or sensitization if not used correctly. By patch testing these products beforehand, individuals can gauge their skin's tolerance and adjust their skincare routine accordingly to minimize the risk of adverse reactions.

In addition to assessing allergic reactions or sensitivities, patch testing can also help identify potential interactions between skincare products. For example, certain combinations of ingredients may be incompatible and could lead to irritation or other adverse effects when used together. Patch testing allows users to identify and avoid such combinations, ensuring the compatibility of their skincare regimen.

While patch testing is an essential precautionary measure, it's essential to interpret the results accurately. Not all reactions indicate an allergy or sensitivity — some degree of redness or irritation may be normal, especially with products containing active ingredients like exfoliants or acne treatments. However, persistent or severe reactions warrant further investigation and may indicate that the product is not suitable for use.

Patch testing is a crucial step in skincare safety, allowing individuals to assess potential allergic reactions or sensitivities before widespread use of a product. By conducting patch tests, users can minimize the risk of adverse reactions and make informed decisions about the products they incorporate into their skincare routine. Whether introducing new products or experimenting with different formulations, patch testing provides a proactive approach to safeguarding skin health and ensuring a positive skincare experience.

By understanding common formulation challenges and embracing the concept of customization, DIY skincare enthusiasts can troubleshoot issues effectively and create personalized skincare products that address their unique needs and preferences with confidence.

Chapter 9

Sustainable Skincare Practices for Eco-Conscious Crafters

As an eco-conscious DIY enthusiast, this chapter empowers you to craft with a conscience. We'll explore sustainable practices that minimize your environmental footprint and contribute to a healthier planet, from sourcing ingredients to choosing packaging.

Selecting organic and fair trade certified ingredients becomes a way to support sustainable farming practices, protect biodiversity, and ensure fair treatment for farmers. Sourcing locally whenever possible reduces transportation emissions, strengthens local economies, and offers greater transparency about ingredient origins. Even foraging or wildcrafting ingredients can be done responsibly – we'll discuss ethical harvesting methods to minimize environmental impact and preserve natural habitats.

Waste reduction is another pillar of sustainable crafting. Simplifying your formulations by focusing on multifunctional ingredients and versatile creations minimizes waste. Embrace the "less is more" philosophy for effective and eco-friendly skincare! Opting for reusable or refillable packaging, like glass jars or silicone pouches, is a simple yet impactful way to ditch single-use plastics and create a more sustainable routine. We'll also explore crafting DIY packaging solutions in small batches to reduce excess inventory and packaging waste, while using creative alternatives like biodegradable paper or fabric wraps.

But sustainability extends beyond your workbench. Researching ingredient suppliers committed to ethical sourcing practices, fair labor standards, and community development initiatives empowers you to make informed choices. We'll delve into ways to engage with local communities and organizations, supporting sustainable development projects, promoting environmental education, and empowering marginalized communities through economic opportunities. Finally, you can become a voice for change by participating in advocacy efforts and supporting organizations working towards environmental conservation, social justice, and sustainable development within the skincare industry and beyond.

By embracing these practices, you'll not only create personal care products that are good for you and the environment, but also contribute to a larger movement for a healthier planet and a more equitable future. So, craft with a conscience and celebrate the beauty of responsible DIY skincare.

9.1

Choosing Ethical and Sustainable Ingredients

Conscious Beauty
The Organic & Fair Trade Choice

In today's fast-paced world, where self-care is as important as ever, the beauty industry is witnessing a transformative shift towards sustainability and ethical sourcing. As consumers become more conscious of the impact their choices have on the planet and its people, there's a growing demand for skincare products that not only deliver results but also align with values of environmental responsibility and social justice.

Organic and fair trade certification has emerged as a beacon of hope in this quest for green glamour. Imagine indulging in luxurious skincare rituals while knowing that every drop and dollop is not just enhancing your beauty but also nurturing the planet and supporting communities worldwide.

Organic certification isn't just about what's not in your skincare—it's about what's in it. By choosing products bearing certifications like USDA Organic or COSMOS Organic, you're embracing ingredients cultivated without synthetic pesticides, herbicides, or fertilizers. It's clean beauty in its purest form, promoting healthier skin and a healthier planet.

But the allure of organic skincare extends beyond its benefits for our complexion. It's a celebration of biodiversity, a commitment to preserving the delicate balance of ecosystems. Organic farming practices prioritize techniques like crop rotation and natural pest control, ensuring that our beauty rituals don't come at the expense of nature's wonders.

And then there's fair trade certification—an invitation to make a difference with every purchase. When you opt for skincare products bearing the Fair Trade Certified label, you're not just pampering your skin—you're empowering farmers and workers in developing countries. Fair trade initiatives ensure fair wages, safe working conditions, and community development projects, fostering a cycle of prosperity and progress.

Transparency and traceability are the cornerstones of the organic and fair trade movement. With certified products, you can trace the journey of every ingredient from farm to formula, knowing that it meets stringent ethical and environmental standards. It's peace of mind in a bottle, allowing you to nourish your skin with confidence and conscience.

By embracing organic and fair trade certification in your skincare routine, you're not just making a statement—you're sparking a revolution. You're redefining beauty as a force for good, where self-care isn't just about looking good but also doing good. So why settle for anything less than green glamour? Transform your skincare routine today and embark on a journey of beauty, sustainability, and social responsibility—one radiant glow at a time.

From Seed to Skin
Local Ingredients for Your DIY Beauty

In a world increasingly conscious of sustainability, a captivating trend is unfolding in the beauty sphere—one that champions the use of locally sourced ingredients in DIY skincare. This movement not only advocates for the health of our skin but also nurtures a profound connection to the land and communities from which these ingredients originate.

At its core, crafting skincare products with locally sourced ingredients embodies the essence of sustainability. When we cultivate our own ingredients or procure them from nearby farms and markets, we minimize the environmental impact associated with transportation and distribution. Picture yourself blending a face mask with homegrown herbs or infusing oils with botanicals harvested from your backyard—each step celebrates the abundance of nature while treading lightly on the planet.

Yet, the allure of DIY skincare extends far beyond its eco-friendly credentials. By engaging in the process of self-production, we forge a deeper connection to the ingredients we use and the communities that produce them. Whether it's whipping up a body scrub with sugar from a local farm or concocting a serum with cold-pressed oils from regional orchards, every creation becomes a testament to our commitment to sustainability and self-sufficiency.

One of the most captivating aspects of DIY skincare is the transparency it affords. With ingredients sourced locally or grown in our own gardens, we have full control over their quality and origins. Imagine crafting a moisturizer with beeswax from a neighboring apiary or infusing a toner with floral waters distilled from blooms cultivated in community gardens—the journey from seed to skincare becomes a story of authenticity and accountability.

From aromatic herbs to nourishing oils, locally sourced ingredients offer a treasure trove of beauty-enhancing benefits. Consider blending a soothing balm with lavender harvested from a nearby field or concocting a facial mist with rosewater distilled from petals grown in your own garden. With each application, we not only nourish our skin but also honor the rich tapestry of botanicals that flourish in our local landscapes.

In conclusion, the movement towards DIY skincare with locally sourced ingredients represents a harmonious blend of sustainability, self-expression, and community connection. By crafting our own beauty treatments with ingredients cultivated close to home, we not only care for our skin but also cultivate a deeper appreciation for the natural world and the communities that sustain it. So let's embrace the art of homemade skincare and embark on a journey of sustainable beauty that's as enriching for the soul as it is for the skin.

Foraged & Found
Sustainable Beauty with Wildcrafted Ingredients

In the realm of skincare, a captivating trend is emerging—one that celebrates the untamed beauty of wildcrafted and foraged ingredients. This movement not only embraces the allure of nature's bounty but also advocates for responsible harvesting practices that honor the environment and preserve natural habitats.

At its heart, wildcrafting and foraging for skincare ingredients represent a deep reverence for the Earth. By venturing into the wilderness or exploring local landscapes, enthusiasts can uncover a treasure trove of botanicals, herbs, and other natural wonders. Imagine strolling through a sun-drenched meadow to gather wild chamomile for a soothing facial steam or trekking through a lush forest to harvest pine needles for an invigorating body scrub. Each excursion becomes a journey of discovery and connection with the natural world.

But the allure of wildcrafted skincare extends beyond its aesthetic appeal. It's about more than just finding beauty in the wild—it's about cultivating a profound sense of stewardship for the environment. Responsible foraging practices, guided by ethical principles, ensure that we minimize our impact on delicate ecosystems and preserve the biodiversity of our surroundings.

For instance, when foraging for seaweed along the coastline, it's essential to harvest only what is needed and to leave behind enough to sustain marine life and coastal ecosystems. Similarly, when gathering wild herbs and flowers, it's crucial to avoid over-harvesting and to respect protected areas and indigenous lands.

One of the most compelling aspects of wildcrafting and foraging for skincare ingredients is the opportunity for connection and communion with nature. Whether it's gathering elderflowers from a sun-dappled meadow or harvesting rose hips from a fragrant hedgerow, each encounter becomes a moment of mindfulness and reverence for the living world around us.

From fragrant blossoms to nutrient-rich greens, wildcrafted and foraged ingredients offer a wealth of beauty-enhancing benefits. Consider infusing oils with wild rose petals for a nourishing facial serum or incorporating foraged berries into a revitalizing face mask. With each creation, we not only nourish our skin but also honor the wisdom of generations past who have long relied on nature's pharmacy for health and healing.

The movement towards wildcrafted and foraged skincare ingredients represents a harmonious blend of beauty, sustainability, and reverence for the natural world. By embracing the practice of ethical foraging, we not only care for our skin but also cultivate a deeper connection with the Earth and its precious ecosystems. So let's venture into the wild and explore the wonders of nature's bounty, one botanical treasure at a time.

9.2

Minimizing Waste and Embracing Zero-Waste Packaging

Less is More
Adopting Minimalist Skincare Formulations

In an era saturated with skincare options, a refreshing trend is emerging—one that prioritizes simplicity and sustainability. It's the movement towards minimalist skincare formulations, where less is truly more. By streamlining ingredients and focusing on multifunctional solutions, this approach not only minimizes waste but also maximizes efficacy, offering a streamlined yet effective skincare routine.

At its essence, minimalist skincare is about paring down formulations to the essentials. By reducing the number of ingredients, we not only simplify our routines but also minimize our environmental footprint. Imagine a moisturizer with just a handful of potent botanical extracts or a cleanser with gentle surfactants derived from natural sources. These minimalist formulations not only deliver results but also reduce the amount of packaging and resources required for production.

But the beauty of minimalist skincare extends beyond its eco-friendly credentials. By focusing on multifunctional ingredients and versatile formulations, we can achieve a myriad of skincare benefits with fewer products. For example, a moisturizer enriched with hyaluronic acid can hydrate and plump the skin while providing antioxidant protection. Similarly, a facial oil infused with vitamin C can brighten and even out skin tone while promoting collagen production.

One of the most compelling aspects of minimalist skincare is its adaptability to individual needs and preferences. Whether you have sensitive skin prone to irritation or a hectic lifestyle that demands simplicity, minimalist formulations offer a tailored approach to skincare that can be customized to suit your unique requirements.

For instance, a minimalist serum formulated with soothing botanicals like chamomile and calendula can provide hydration and calming benefits for sensitive skin types. Alternatively, a lightweight gel moisturizer with hyaluronic acid and niacinamide can offer hydration and oil control for those with combination or oily skin.

In conclusion, the movement towards minimalist skincare formulations represents a holistic approach to beauty that prioritizes simplicity, efficacy, and sustainability. By embracing fewer ingredients and versatile formulations, we not only streamline our routines but also minimize our environmental impact and maximize our skincare benefits. So let's simplify our skincare rituals and discover the beauty of less—because when it comes to skincare, sometimes, less truly is more.

Sustainable Solutions
Choosing Reusable and Refillable Packaging

In a world grappling with plastic pollution, a growing number of skincare enthusiasts are championing a sustainable solution: reusable and refillable packaging. By opting for alternatives like glass jars, aluminum tins, or silicone pouches, these eco-conscious consumers are not only reducing single-use plastic waste but also paving the way for a more planet-friendly approach to beauty.

At its core, the choice of packaging material plays a pivotal role in determining the environmental impact of skincare products. By steering clear of single-use plastics and embracing reusable or refillable options, we can significantly decrease the amount of waste destined for landfills and oceans.

Imagine a moisturizer housed in a sleek glass jar that can be endlessly refilled or a cleanser packaged in a sturdy aluminum tin that can be repurposed or recycled. These alternatives not only minimize our carbon footprint but also add a touch of elegance to our skincare routines.

But the benefits of reusable and refillable packaging extend beyond environmental considerations. By investing in durable containers that can be used again and again, we're not only reducing waste but also saving money in the long run. It's a win-win situation that aligns with both our ethical values and our practical needs.

One of the most compelling aspects of reusable and refillable packaging is its versatility. Whether you prefer the classic charm of glass jars, the lightweight convenience of aluminum tins, or the flexibility of silicone pouches, there's an option to suit every taste and lifestyle.

For instance, a skincare brand might offer its products in refillable glass bottles that can be returned and replenished at designated refill stations. Alternatively, consumers might opt for silicone pouches that can be easily squeezed and reused, reducing the need for additional packaging materials.

In conclusion, the movement towards reusable and refillable skincare packaging represents a significant step towards a more sustainable and conscientious approach to beauty. By choosing alternatives to single-use plastics, we not only reduce our environmental impact but also set a precedent for a greener future. So let's embrace reusable and refillable options and embark on a journey towards a more beautiful—and sustainable—world.

Crafted with Care
DIY Packaging Solutions for Homemade Skincare

A wave of eco-consciousness is sweeping through, driving enthusiasts towards a more sustainable path. In this movement, DIY skincare aficionados stand out for their innovative approach not only in crafting products but also in packaging them sustainably. Let's delve into the world of DIY packaging solutions, where creativity meets environmental responsibility.

At the heart of DIY skincare lies the ethos of crafting with purpose. By creating products in small batches, enthusiasts not only ensure freshness and potency but also reduce excess inventory and packaging waste. Picture blending a revitalizing facial serum in a reusable glass dropper bottle or whipping up a nourishing body butter stored in a refillable aluminum tin. These minimalist choices not only prioritize sustainability but also elevate the overall skincare experience.

In the quest for sustainable packaging, DIYers are exploring alternative materials that minimize environmental impact. For instance, crafting biodegradable paper pouches to package herbal bath salts or using fabric wraps made from organic cotton to encase handmade soap bars. These eco-friendly alternatives not only reduce the reliance on single-use plastics but also add a personal touch to homemade skincare products, enhancing their appeal while minimizing ecological footprint.

One of the hallmarks of DIY packaging solutions is their ability to marry aesthetic appeal with environmental consciousness. From hand-stamped labels made from recycled paper to intricately knotted jute twine securing eco-friendly lip balm tubes, every detail is thoughtfully designed to enhance the presentation of homemade skincare products while minimizing waste. These visually appealing packages serve as a testament to the creator's commitment to sustainability and conscious consumption.

DIY packaging solutions offer unparalleled versatility and customization, allowing creators to tailor packaging to their individual needs and preferences. For example, repurposing glass jars salvaged from food containers to store homemade facial masks or opting for compostable cellulose bags to package exfoliating scrubs. By embracing creativity and resourcefulness, DIYers not only reduce their environmental footprint but also showcase the beauty of sustainable living.

DIY packaging solutions represent a powerful step towards a more sustainable future for skincare. By embracing creativity, ingenuity, and environmental responsibility, DIY enthusiasts are crafting a greener world, one package at a time. Let's celebrate their dedication to sustainability and join them in their journey towards a more eco-friendly approach to beauty.

9.3

Supporting Fair Trade and Community Initiatives

Building Bridges
Ethical Sourcing in Skincare Supply Chains

A quiet revolution is taking place—one that prioritizes ethics and responsibility in the sourcing of ingredients. This movement, focused on ethical supply chains, emphasizes the importance of researching suppliers and manufacturers committed to fair labor standards, sustainable practices, and community development initiatives. Let's explore why ethical sourcing matters and how it's shaping the future of skincare.

At its core, ethical skincare begins with a profound respect for every ingredient's journey. This means delving deep into the origins of each component, from the fields where plants are grown to the hands that harvest and process them. For instance, seeking out suppliers who support fair trade practices ensures that farmers receive fair compensation for their labor, empowering communities and fostering economic stability.

Fair labor standards are non-negotiable in ethical skincare. By partnering with manufacturers who uphold fair labor practices, skincare brands uphold the dignity and rights of workers. From ensuring safe working conditions to advocating for living wages, ethical sourcing prioritizes the well-being of those who contribute to the creation of skincare products.

Ethical skincare isn't just about sourcing ingredients—it's about nurturing communities. Brands committed to ethical sourcing invest in initiatives that uplift and empower local communities, from education and healthcare projects to sustainable development programs. By supporting community growth and prosperity, ethical skincare brands create positive change that extends far beyond the beauty industry.

Transparency is key in ethical skincare. By providing consumers with insight into their sourcing practices, brands build trust and accountability. Whether through certifications, sourcing stories, or supply chain transparency reports, ethical skincare brands empower consumers to make informed choices and support responsible practices.

In conclusion, ethical sourcing is not just a trend—it's a fundamental shift in the way we approach skincare. By prioritizing fair labor, sustainable practices, and community development, ethical skincare brands set a new standard for beauty—one that values integrity, compassion, and responsibility. As consumers, we have the power to shape this movement by supporting brands that prioritize ethics and sustainability. Let's embrace the ethos of ethical skincare and pave the way for a more beautiful, equitable, and sustainable future.

Fostering Change
Skincare's Role in Community Engagement

In the ever-evolving landscape of skincare, a vital aspect gaining momentum is community engagement. Beyond just products, brands are stepping up to engage with local communities and organizations, championing sustainable development projects, promoting environmental education, and empowering marginalized groups through economic opportunities. Let's delve into why community engagement matters and how skincare is making a difference.

Community engagement in skincare transcends mere transactions. It's about forging meaningful connections with the communities where ingredients are sourced, products are made, and consumers reside. By engaging directly with local communities, skincare brands not only gain insight into their needs but also foster partnerships that drive positive change.

Skincare brands are increasingly investing in sustainable development projects that benefit local communities and the environment. Whether it's funding reforestation efforts in regions affected by deforestation or supporting clean water initiatives in areas facing scarcity, these projects aim to create a lasting impact on both people and the planet.

Environmental education lies at the heart of community engagement in skincare. Brands are taking proactive steps to raise awareness about sustainability issues, such as plastic pollution, climate change, and biodiversity loss. Through workshops, campaigns, and educational materials, skincare brands empower consumers to make informed choices and take action for a greener future.

One of the most significant impacts of community engagement in skincare is its ability to empower marginalized groups through economic opportunities. By partnering with local cooperatives, women's groups, and indigenous communities, skincare brands create pathways for economic empowerment and social inclusion. From sourcing ingredients to manufacturing products, these collaborations uplift communities and foster resilience.

Community engagement is not just a buzzword—it's a driving force behind positive change in the skincare industry. By engaging with local communities, supporting sustainable development projects, promoting environmental education, and empowering marginalized groups, skincare brands are making a tangible difference in the world. As consumers, we have the power to support these efforts by choosing brands that prioritize community engagement and social responsibility. Together, we can foster a more equitable, sustainable, and beautiful future for all.

The Power of Choice
How You Can Change the Skincare Industry

In today's interconnected world, consumers are increasingly recognizing the power of advocacy and activism in driving positive change. This sentiment holds true in the skincare industry, where a growing number of individuals are not only seeking products for their skin but also for their values. From environmental conservation to social justice and sustainable development, advocacy efforts are shaping the skincare landscape and beyond.

Participating in advocacy efforts within the skincare industry involves raising awareness about pressing issues such as plastic pollution, deforestation, and fair labor practices. It's about amplifying voices and mobilizing action to address systemic challenges that impact both people and the planet. Through social media campaigns, petitions, and grassroots initiatives, individuals are leveraging their influence to spark meaningful change.

Supporting organizations dedicated to environmental conservation, social justice, and sustainable development is another crucial aspect of advocacy in the skincare industry. By aligning with nonprofits, NGOs, and grassroots movements, individuals can contribute to collective efforts aimed at protecting ecosystems, advocating for marginalized communities, and promoting ethical business practices. Whether through donations, volunteer work, or collaboration, every contribution makes a difference in the fight for a better world.

Environmental conservation is a key focus area for advocacy and activism in the skincare industry. With growing concerns about climate change and biodiversity loss, consumers are increasingly demanding products that minimize their ecological footprint. This has led to a rise in eco-friendly skincare brands that prioritize sustainable sourcing, packaging, and manufacturing practices. By supporting these brands and advocating for stronger environmental regulations, individuals can help protect precious natural resources for future generations.

Social justice is another critical issue driving advocacy in the skincare industry. From fair wages and working conditions to racial and gender equality, consumers are pushing for greater accountability and transparency throughout the supply chain. By advocating for diversity and inclusion in the beauty industry and supporting brands that prioritize ethical labor practices, individuals can help create a more just and equitable world.

Sustainable development is at the core of advocacy and activism in the skincare industry. By promoting economic growth, social inclusion, and environmental protection, individuals can contribute to building a more sustainable future for all. This includes supporting initiatives that empower marginalized communities, promote renewable energy, and foster innovation in sustainable technologies. Through collective action, we can create a world where skincare is not just about looking good but also doing good.

Advocacy and activism play a vital role in shaping the skincare industry and driving positive change in the world. By participating in advocacy efforts and supporting organizations working to promote environmental conservation, social justice, and sustainable development, individuals can make a meaningful impact. Together, we can build a more ethical, equitable, and sustainable future for the skincare industry and beyond.

By embracing sustainable skincare practices, eco-conscious crafters can not only create healthier, more eco-friendly skincare products but also contribute to broader efforts to protect the planet and promote social and economic equity.

Chapter 10

Sharing Your Passion for Natural Skincare

Have you ever considered sharing your passion for DIY natural skincare? This chapter ignites the joy of inspiring others! From hosting workshops to gifting homemade creations, we'll explore ways to empower those around you to embrace a natural approach to beauty.

Imagine hosting hands-on workshops – a space to share basic formulation techniques, swap skincare recipes, and foster a spirit of creativity with friends, family, or even community groups. Collaborate with local yoga studios, wellness centers, or farmers' markets to expand your reach and connect with diverse audiences. Knowledge is power, so consider volunteering your expertise to lead workshops for underserved communities, schools, or youth organizations, promoting skincare education and self-care practices.

The gift of homemade skincare is truly special. Create personalized sets for birthdays, holidays, or celebrations! Combine your creations with thoughtful packaging and educational materials to elevate the experience. Let your gifts reflect your values – explore sustainable options like reusable containers, biodegradable wrapping paper, or plantable packaging for a beautiful and eco-conscious touch. Don't forget the finishing touch! Design custom labels and branding that reflect your unique style, adding a personal touch and showcasing your dedication to the craft.

The online world offers a fantastic platform for connection. Share your DIY journey, formulations, and tips on social media to connect with fellow enthusiasts and inspire others to explore natural skincare. Join online forums or communities dedicated to DIY skincare – a space to share knowledge, participate in discussions, and seek advice from experienced crafters. Feeling ambitious? Start a skincare blog or YouTube channel! Document your projects, review ingredients, and provide tutorials and troubleshooting tips. This is a fantastic way to build a valuable resource for fellow enthusiasts and establish yourself as a knowledgeable voice in the community.

By sharing your passion through workshops, thoughtful gifts, and online engagement, you'll not only inspire others to embark on their own DIY skincare journeys, but also cultivate a sense of connection and empowerment within the natural skincare community. So, spread the love and celebrate the joy of sharing your passion for creating personalized, natural skincare solutions.

10.1

DIY Skincare Workshops and Community Events

Crafting Connections
Hosting DIY Skincare Workshops

Carving out moments for meaningful connections and self-care is essential. Hosting hands-on DIY skincare workshops provides a unique opportunity to gather friends, family, or community members and embark on a journey of exploration and self-discovery. By involving a diverse group of individuals in these workshops, hosts can create an enriching experience that fosters creativity, camaraderie, and empowerment.

When considering who to involve in DIY skincare workshops, the possibilities are endless. Friends looking for a fun and educational activity to share, family members seeking a bonding experience, or members of a community group interested in holistic wellness—all can benefit from participating in these workshops. By bringing together individuals with varied backgrounds, interests, and perspectives, hosts create a dynamic environment ripe for learning and collaboration.

At the heart of hosting DIY skincare workshops lies the desire to empower participants with knowledge and practical skills. By teaching basic formulation techniques and sharing skincare recipes, hosts equip participants with the tools they need to create their own personalized skincare products. Whether it's crafting nourishing body butters, refreshing facial masks, or soothing lip balms, participants learn to harness the power of natural ingredients to care for their skin in a holistic and sustainable way.

Beyond the act of formulation, DIY skincare workshops offer a space for connection and community building. As participants collaborate on recipes, share skincare tips, and bond over a shared love for natural beauty, meaningful relationships are formed. These workshops provide an opportunity for individuals to come together, support one another, and celebrate the joys of self-care in a supportive and inclusive environment.

Moreover, hosting DIY skincare workshops offers an opportunity to promote environmental consciousness and sustainability. By emphasizing the use of natural, eco-friendly ingredients and minimizing packaging waste, hosts inspire participants to adopt more environmentally friendly skincare practices. This focus on sustainability not only benefits the planet but also encourages participants to make mindful choices that prioritize their own well-being and the health of the environment.

Hosting DIY skincare workshops is a powerful way to nurture creativity, connection, and community. By involving friends, family, or community members in these workshops, hosts create an enriching experience that empowers participants to take control of their skincare routines and embrace natural beauty in a sustainable and inclusive way. So why not gather your loved ones or community members and embark on a journey of exploration and self-discovery through the world of DIY skincare? The connections you'll make and the memories you'll create will be truly priceless.

Strengthening Communities
Collaborating with Local Businesses

In the realm of holistic wellness and self-care, collaboration is key to creating vibrant and thriving communities. Partnering with local businesses such as yoga studios, wellness centers, or farmers' markets to offer skincare workshops can be a powerful way to expand your reach, engage with diverse audiences, and foster connections within the community. Let's explore the benefits of these collaborations and how they can enrich both your workshops and the local community.

When it comes to hosting skincare workshops, collaborating with local businesses opens up a world of opportunities. By partnering with establishments that share a similar ethos of wellness and sustainability, hosts can tap into existing networks and reach new audiences who are already interested in holistic health and self-care. This allows for greater visibility and exposure, attracting participants who may not have otherwise been aware of the workshops.

Yoga studios, wellness centers, and farmers' markets are natural partners for skincare workshops, as they often attract individuals who prioritize health, wellness, and sustainability. By offering skincare workshops as part of their programming, these businesses can enhance the overall experience for their clients and customers, providing valuable opportunities for learning and self-improvement in addition to their core offerings.

Moreover, collaborating with local businesses allows hosts to tap into the expertise and resources of their partners. For example, hosting workshops at a yoga studio may provide access to dedicated space for activities and events, while partnering with a farmers' market may offer opportunities to source fresh, locally grown ingredients for skincare formulations. These collaborations enrich the workshop experience and enhance the quality of the products created.

From a community perspective, partnering with local businesses fosters a sense of connection and support within the neighborhood. By working together towards a common goal of promoting health, wellness, and sustainability, hosts and their partners can strengthen relationships with customers, clients, and community members, creating a ripple effect of positive impact that extends beyond the workshops themselves.

Collaborating with local businesses to offer skincare workshops is a win-win for hosts, partners, and the community at large. By expanding your reach, engaging with diverse audiences, and tapping into the resources of your partners, you can create enriching experiences that promote holistic wellness and strengthen community connections. So why not reach out to your local yoga studio, wellness center, or farmers' market and explore the possibilities of collaboration? Together, you can create something truly special for your community.

Empowering Through Education
Community Outreach Skincare Workshops

In the pursuit of holistic wellness and empowerment, skincare education plays a vital role. Community outreach initiatives that involve volunteering time and expertise to lead skincare workshops for underserved communities, schools, or youth organizations are a powerful way to promote skincare education and self-care practices. Let's delve into the importance of these workshops and the impact they have on individuals and communities.

At the heart of community outreach skincare workshops is the belief that everyone deserves access to knowledge and resources that promote self-care and well-being. By volunteering time and expertise to lead these workshops, hosts empower individuals in underserved communities to take control of their skincare routines and prioritize their health.

Underserved communities, schools, and youth organizations often face barriers to accessing skincare education and resources. By bringing skincare workshops directly to these communities, hosts break down these barriers and create opportunities for learning and growth. Participants gain valuable skills and knowledge that can have a lasting impact on their health and confidence.

Skincare workshops in underserved communities serve as a platform for promoting self-care practices and instilling a sense of empowerment. Participants learn basic skincare techniques, gain insight into the importance of skincare ingredients, and discover affordable and accessible ways to care for their skin. This knowledge not only improves their physical well-being but also boosts their self-esteem and confidence.

Moreover, community outreach skincare workshops foster a sense of connection and support within the communities they serve. By volunteering time and expertise, hosts demonstrate a commitment to uplifting others and giving back to their communities. Participants feel valued and supported, knowing that someone cares about their health and well-being.

From a broader perspective, community outreach skincare workshops contribute to promoting health equity and social justice. By providing access to skincare education and resources in underserved communities, hosts address disparities in healthcare and empower individuals to advocate for their own health needs. This grassroots approach to wellness promotes a more equitable and inclusive society for all.

In conclusion, community outreach skincare workshops are a powerful tool for promoting skincare education and self-care practices in underserved communities. By volunteering time and expertise to lead these workshops, hosts empower individuals to prioritize their health and well-being, fostering a sense of empowerment and resilience. Together, we can create healthier, happier communities where everyone has the opportunity to thrive.

10.2

Gift Ideas
and Packaging Inspiration

Handcrafted Beauty
Elevating Gift-Giving with DIY Skincare Sets

In a world where personal connections often get lost amidst the sea of commercialized products, DIY skincare gift sets stand out as tokens of genuine care and thoughtfulness. These bespoke creations offer a unique opportunity to express love and creativity on special occasions like birthdays, holidays, or bridal showers.

At the core of DIY skincare sets is the essence of customization. Crafting products from scratch enables creators to select ingredients, scents, and textures tailored to the recipient's preferences. Whether it's a luxurious body butter or a refreshing lip balm, each item exudes individuality and affection.

Packaging plays a vital role in enhancing the gift-giving experience, adding an extra layer of charm and anticipation. Thoughtfully presented in rustic kraft boxes or adorned with delicate labels, these sets capture the essence of heartfelt gestures.

Beyond their aesthetic appeal, DIY skincare sets offer an educational journey, empowering recipients with skincare tips and insights. Sustainable and eco-friendly, these sets align with ethical gift-giving practices, showcasing a commitment to conscious living.

In essence, DIY skincare gift sets transcend materialism—they're expressions of love, creativity, and wellness. They invite recipients to indulge in a pampering experience that nourishes both body and soul, making them the perfect embodiment of handcrafted beauty in a commercialized world.

Here are some examples of DIY skincare gift sets that you can create:

Pampering Spa Set: This set can include a homemade sugar scrub, a soothing bath soak, and a moisturizing body butter. Package them in a pretty basket or a reusable jar, along with a loofah or a bath sponge for added luxury.

Facial Care Kit: Create a set tailored for facial care, including a gentle facial cleanser, a hydrating face mist, and a nourishing facial oil or serum. Pair it with a soft facial towel or a skincare brush for a complete skincare experience.

Lip Care Duo: For those who love lip care, assemble a set featuring a homemade lip scrub to exfoliate and a lip balm to hydrate and protect. Present them in a cute tin or a small pouch, perfect for on-the-go lip care.

Natural Beauty Essentials: Curate a collection of essential skincare products, such as a multipurpose balm for dry patches, a refreshing toner, and a versatile oil blend for face, body, and hair. Package them in reusable glass bottles or jars for an eco-friendly touch.

Hand Care Set: Craft a set focused on hand care, including a nourishing hand scrub, a moisturizing hand cream, and a cuticle oil for healthy nails. Present them in a decorative box or a woven basket, alongside a nail file or hand towel.

Soothing Sensitive Skin Kit: Prepare a set tailored for sensitive skin, featuring gentle and calming products like a soothing oatmeal bath soak, a calming facial mask, and a hydrating aloe vera gel. Package them in minimalist glass jars for a clean and elegant look.

DIY Face Mask Trio: Create a trio of homemade face masks targeting different skin concerns, such as detoxifying clay mask, a hydrating honey mask, and a brightening citrus mask. Package them in small jars or tubes, along with a brush for easy application.

Remember to personalize the gift sets based on the recipient's preferences and skincare needs, and don't forget to include instructions or tips on how to use each product for the best results.

Green Glamour
Eco-Friendly Packaging for All Ages

Ladies and girls, picture this: skincare products that not only make you look good but also make you feel good about your impact on the planet. That's where eco-friendly packaging steps in, blending beauty with environmental consciousness in a way that resonates with women of all ages.

Imagine reaching for your favorite moisturizer housed in a chic glass jar. Not only does it exude luxury, but it's also reusable, promoting a circular economy that's as stylish as it is sustainable. For the younger crowd, it's about embracing a lifestyle that values quality over quantity, while for the seasoned ladies, it's a nod to the timeless elegance of classic beauty.

Now, let's talk wrapping. Biodegradable paper, made from recycled materials or plant fibers, offers a guilt-free alternative to traditional packaging. It's compostable, recyclable, and adds a touch of eco-chic to your beauty routine. From millennials striving for a zero-waste lifestyle to mature women championing sustainability, it's a packaging choice that speaks volumes about your values.

But here's where it gets really exciting—plantable packaging. Yes, you heard that right. Picture opening your skincare product to find seeds embedded in the packaging. Plant them, water them, and watch them bloom into vibrant flowers. It's a beautiful reminder of the cycle of renewal and regeneration, appealing to women of all ages who appreciate the beauty of nature.

So, whether you're in your twenties or your golden years, eco-friendly packaging in skincare is a trend that's here to stay. It's about more than just looking good—it's about feeling good, knowing that your beauty routine is making a positive impact on the planet. Let's embrace green glamour and pave the way for a more sustainable future, one package at a time.

Personalized Beauty
Custom Labels and Branding for Your Creations

In the realm of skincare, presentation holds immense significance. It's not merely about the products you concoct but equally about how you showcase them to the world. Enter custom labels and branding materials—a game-changer in the DIY skincare landscape. These personalized touches not only enhance the presentation of your homemade skincare products but also serve as reflections of your unique style and values, enriching the gifting experience for your loved ones.

Imagine receiving a jar of homemade body butter, adorned with a label bearing your name or a whimsical design that perfectly encapsulates your essence. It's more than skincare—it's an expression of artistry and care. Custom labels allow you to infuse your products with a touch of luxury and individuality, setting them apart from mass-produced alternatives.

But beyond aesthetics, custom labels enable storytelling. They narrate the journey of your skincare creations, spotlighting the ingredients you carefully select, the processes you meticulously follow, and the principles you hold dear. Each element adds depth and meaning to your products, resonating with customers who share your values.

Now, let's delve into the practical aspect—the creation process. Several software, apps, and online services offer user-friendly platforms for designing custom labels. Tools like Canva, Adobe Spark, and Avery Design & Print provide a plethora of templates, graphics, and fonts to bring your label visions to life. Moreover, online printing services such as Vistaprint and Sticker Mule offer high-quality printing options for your labels, ensuring professional results.

And when it comes to branding materials, consider incorporating your custom labels into packaging, business cards, and thank-you notes. Websites like Moo and Zazzle offer customizable options for various branding materials, allowing you to maintain consistency across your skincare line.

Custom labels and branding materials serve as the finishing touch that elevates your skincare creations, making them not just products but experiences. With the plethora of design tools and printing services available, there's no limit to the creativity and personalization you can infuse into your skincare brand. So, let your imagination soar, and watch as your skincare creations become a reflection of your unique identity and values.

10.3

Building a Supportive Skincare Community Online

Fostering Digital Connections
Share Your Skincare Journey

In today's digitally connected world, the internet has become a powerful tool for building communities around shared interests and passions. Skincare enthusiasts are no exception, as they flock to social media platforms like Instagram, YouTube, and Pinterest to connect with others who share their love for all things skincare. In this digital landscape, fostering a supportive skincare community online has become not only feasible but also incredibly rewarding.

One of the first steps in building a supportive skincare community online is choosing the right platform. Different social media platforms offer unique features and cater to different audiences, so it's essential to select the one that best aligns with your goals and communication style. Whether you prefer the visual appeal of Instagram, the educational format of YouTube, or the inspiration-driven nature of Pinterest, there's a platform out there for you to share your skincare journey.

Authenticity is paramount when it comes to building a supportive community online. Sharing your skincare journey, including both the highs and lows, helps to establish trust and relatability with your audience. By being transparent about your experiences with different products and formulations, you can create a space where others feel comfortable sharing their own skincare struggles and triumphs.

Engaging content is also key to keeping your audience interested and invested in your skincare community. From sharing skincare tips and DIY recipes to providing product reviews and educational resources, there are countless ways to add value to your followers' skincare journey. Visual content such as photos and videos can enhance your messaging and make it more engaging for your audience.

Connecting with fellow skincare enthusiasts is another essential aspect of building a supportive online community. By engaging with other creators and followers within your niche, you can foster relationships and collaborations that enrich the overall experience for everyone involved. Supporting others in the community not only strengthens your network but also creates a sense of camaraderie among fellow skincare enthusiasts.

As you share your knowledge and expertise with your audience, remember to inspire and educate others about the benefits of natural skincare. Empowering your followers to make informed choices about their skincare routines and products is a powerful way to foster a sense of community and camaraderie. By providing valuable insights and resources, you can help others on their skincare journey while also reinforcing your position as a trusted authority in the skincare space.

Encouraging interaction and dialogue among your followers is crucial for fostering a sense of community and engagement. By asking questions, creating polls, and inviting feedback, you can spark meaningful conversations that deepen connections and encourage participation. Responding promptly to comments and messages demonstrates that you value your followers' input and encourages them to continue engaging with your content.

Sharing user-generated content from your followers is another effective way to showcase the impact of your skincare community. By reposting photos, testimonials, and reviews from satisfied customers and fans, you can highlight the positive experiences and contributions of your community members. This not only reinforces the sense of community but also serves as social proof of the value and efficacy of your skincare products and content.

Cultivating a positive and inclusive environment within your skincare community is essential for fostering trust and loyalty among your followers. By monitoring comments and interactions and taking proactive steps to address any negativity or toxicity, you can create a safe and supportive space where everyone feels welcome and respected. Reinforcing values of kindness, empathy, and acceptance helps to nurture a culture of positivity and mutual support within your community.

Consistency and authenticity are key principles to keep in mind as you build and nurture your skincare community online. By staying true to your brand voice and values and consistently delivering valuable content that resonates with your audience, you can build trust and credibility over time. Authenticity builds connections and fosters loyalty among your followers, so be genuine and transparent in your interactions and messaging.

Finally, measuring success and adjusting strategies based on feedback and data is essential for optimizing your engagement efforts and maximizing your impact. Monitoring social media metrics such as likes, comments, shares, and follower growth can provide valuable insights into the effectiveness of your content and engagement strategies. Use this data to refine your approach and tailor your content to better meet the needs and preferences of your audience.

Building a supportive skincare community online requires a combination of authenticity, engagement, and value-driven content. By leveraging social media platforms to share your skincare journey, formulations, and tips, you can connect with fellow DIY enthusiasts and inspire others to explore natural skincare. Building a thriving online community takes time and effort, but the rewards of sharing knowledge, fostering connections, and empowering others are well worth it.

Nurturing Community
The Value of Online Forums in DIY Skincare

In the vast landscape of the internet, there exists a thriving community of individuals passionate about crafting their own skincare products. At the heart of this community lie online forums, Facebook groups, and subreddit communities dedicated to DIY skincare. These digital spaces serve as gathering grounds for enthusiasts from all walks of life, united by a shared love for natural skincare and a desire to learn, create, and connect.

Participating in online forums offers a myriad of benefits for DIY skincare enthusiasts. For example, platforms like Reddit's "r/ DIYBeauty" subreddit provide a space for members to discuss a wide range of skincare topics, from formulating recipes to troubleshooting common issues. Similarly, Facebook groups such as "DIY Skincare Enthusiasts" foster lively discussions and provide a supportive environment for sharing experiences and seeking advice.

Beyond knowledge sharing, online forums provide a sense of community and support that is often invaluable on the DIY skincare path. Take, for instance, the "Skincare Addiction" subreddit, which boasts over 1.6 million members. Here, individuals from around the world come together to celebrate successes, commiserate over setbacks, and offer encouragement to fellow skincare enthusiasts.

Moreover, engaging in online forums sparks inspiration and creativity. Platforms like "The Skincare Addiction" subreddit frequently feature posts showcasing members' latest skincare creations, from homemade serums to luxurious body butters. Seeing the innovative formulations and creative packaging ideas shared by others inspires individuals to experiment and push the boundaries of their own skincare craft.

Critically, online forums also serve as platforms for feedback and advice. For instance, the "DIY Beauty" forum on Reddit allows members to post their formulations for critique and feedback from the community. Whether seeking input on ingredient substitutions, troubleshooting texture issues, or verifying the potency of a formulation, the collective wisdom of the community provides invaluable guidance.

Furthermore, online forums offer networking opportunities, connecting individuals with like-minded enthusiasts, ingredient suppliers, and potential collaborators. For example, forums like "Skincare Talk" on Makeupalley.com provide a space for members to share recommendations for trusted ingredient suppliers and discuss sourcing strategies.

Online forums play a vital role in nurturing the DIY skincare community, providing a space for knowledge sharing, community building, inspiration, feedback, and networking. By actively participating in these virtual communities, enthusiasts can enrich their skincare journey, expand their knowledge, and forge meaningful connections with fellow crafters. Ultimately, it's the sense of belonging and camaraderie fostered within these online forums that makes them indispensable to the DIY skincare experience.

Crafting Connections
The Power of Blogging and Content Creation

Starting a skincare blog or YouTube channel to share DIY projects, review skincare ingredients, and offer tutorials and troubleshooting tips is a fantastic way to connect with fellow skincare enthusiasts and build a valuable resource for the community. However, before diving into the world of content creation, it's essential to consider the various steps involved and the platforms available to showcase your expertise.

Firstly, defining your niche is crucial. Decide what aspect of skincare you're most passionate about and what sets you apart from other content creators. Are you interested in creating DIY skincare recipes, providing in-depth ingredient reviews, sharing skincare routines, or offering tips and tricks for addressing common skincare concerns? Narrowing down your focus will help you attract a targeted audience and establish yourself as an authority in your chosen niche.

Once you've determined your niche, you'll need to choose the right platform to showcase your content. For written content, starting a blog using platforms like WordPress, Blogger, or Squarespace is a popular choice. These platforms offer customizable templates, easy-to-use interfaces, and the flexibility to create and organize written content effectively. Additionally, blogging platforms often provide built-in features for search engine optimization (SEO), allowing you to increase your blog's visibility and attract organic traffic.

If you prefer visual content, creating a YouTube channel may be more suitable. YouTube provides a platform for sharing video tutorials, product reviews, skincare routines, and other engaging content. With its vast audience and search capabilities, YouTube offers immense potential for reaching a broad audience and building a loyal following. You can also leverage YouTube's monetization features, such as ads and sponsorships, to generate income from your content.

In addition to blogs and YouTube, social media platforms like Instagram, Pinterest, and TikTok can complement your main platform and help you reach a wider audience. Instagram, with its visual nature, is ideal for sharing skincare routines, product recommendations, and behind-the-scenes content. Pinterest is excellent for curating inspiration boards, sharing DIY recipes, and driving traffic to your blog or YouTube channel. TikTok offers a fun and engaging platform for creating short-form video content and showcasing your personality and creativity.

When it comes to naming some useful platforms, WordPress stands out as one of the most popular blogging platforms, offering a user-friendly interface, customizable themes, and a wide range of plugins to enhance functionality. Blogger, owned by Google, is another option known for its simplicity and integration with other Google services. Squarespace is a versatile platform that combines website building and blogging capabilities, making it suitable for beginners and advanced users alike.

For video content creation, YouTube is the go-to platform, providing robust editing tools, analytics, and monetization options. Vimeo is an alternative platform known for its high-quality video hosting and customizable player options, catering to filmmakers, artists, and content creators. Additionally, social media platforms like Instagram, Pinterest, and TikTok offer opportunities for sharing visual content and engaging with your audience in creative ways.

Ultimately, the key to success in skincare blogging and content creation lies in delivering valuable and engaging content that resonates with your audience. By leveraging the right platforms and consistently providing high-quality content, you can build a loyal following, establish yourself as a trusted source of skincare information, and contribute positively to the skincare community.

By sharing your passion for natural skincare through workshops, gifts, and online communities, you can not only inspire others to embark on their own DIY skincare journey but also foster a sense of connection and empowerment within the skincare community.

Epilogue

Thank you for embarking on this natural beauty journey with me through the pages of "DIY Natural Skincare." I hope you have found inspiration, knowledge, and joy in creating your personalized beauty products.

Your feedback is invaluable. I invite you to leave an honest review of the book. Your words will not only help other readers discover the benefits of natural skincare but also allow me to improve and provide even more useful content.

For additional resources, recipes, and tips, visit our website at www.craftyourbetterself.com. Continue to explore, experiment, and enjoy the wonderful world of natural skincare.

With gratitude and wishes for radiant skin,

Eleanor Greene